Biopsy Pathology of the Oesophagus, Stomach and Duodenum

Biopsy Pathology of the Oesophagus, Stomach and Duodenum

D. W. DAY
MB, BChir, MRCPath, MA(Cantab)
Senior Lecturer in Pathology
University of Liverpool
and Honorary Consultant Pathologist
Royal Liverpool Hospital

with a contribution by

O. A. N. HUSAIN
MD, FRCPath
Consultant Pathologist
Cytology Department,
St Stephen's Hospital and Charing Cross Hospital
London

A WILEY MEDICAL PUBLICATION

JOHN WILEY & SONS
New York

*Published in the USA
by Wiley Medical, a Division of
John Wiley & Sons, Inc., New York*

© *1986 D. W. Day*

ISBN 0–471–01046–4

Printed in Great Britain

*Library of Congress Catalog
Card No. 85–20279*

Library of Congress Cataloging-in-Publication Data

Day, D. W., 1944–
  Biopsy pathology of the oesophagus, stomach, and duodenum.

  (Biopsy pathology series) (A Wiley medical publication)
  Includes bibliographies and index.
  1. Esophagus—Biopsy.   2. Stomach—Biopsy.
3. Duodenum—Biopsy.   4. Digestive organs—Diseases—
Diagnosis.   I. Husain, O. A. N.   II. Title.   III. Series.
IV. Series: Wiley medical publication.   [DNLM:
1. Duodenal Diseases—pathology.   2. Esophageal Diseases
—pathology.   3. Stomach Diseases—pathology.
WI 100 D273b]
RC804.B5D39   1986   616.3'0758   85–20279
ISBN 0–471–01046–4

Contents

Preface

Biopsies from the upper gastrointestinal tract form an increasing proportion of a histopathologist's workload, a direct result of the introduction and escalating use of fibre-optic endoscopy. The purpose of this book is to illustrate, describe and discuss the significance of the light microscopic appearances of the more common and important conditions affecting the mucosa of the oesophagus, stomach and duodenum likely to be met with in clinical practice. I have included as well, where appropriate, brief descriptions of endoscopic appearances since 'what the endoscopist saw' is a vital component in the diagnostic process.

Electron microscopy and immunohistochemical techniques are sometimes necessary and occasionally crucial adjuncts in diagnosis, and although the emphasis in this book is on light microscopy, indications for these more specialized procedures are mentioned in the text.

Cytology of the oesophagus, stomach and duodenum is not as widely practised as it should be. I see it as a complementary technique to biopsy which in particular circumstances, notably pre-cancerous conditions such as tylosis, Barrett's oesophagus, pernicious anaemia and in operated stomach patients, is more likely to detect malignant or pre-malignant changes than random biopsies alone. I have been fortunate in having Dr Husain's valuable contribution on the cytology of the upper gastrointestinal tract (Chapter 14).

I am indebted to the following colleagues who kindly provided material for illustration: Dr A. E. Bishop, Dr A. J. Blackshaw, Dr C. T. Burrow, Professor M. Crespi, Professor K. Elster, Dr T. R. Helliwell, Professor P. G. Isaacson and the Editor of *Histopathology* for permission to reproduce Figs 7.1 and 7.2, Dr J. R. Jass, Dr W. Kenyon, Professor S-C. Ming, Dr B. C. Morson, Dr N. Munoz, Dr J. R. G. Nash, Dr J. Piris, Professor J. M. Polak, Dr A. B. Price, Dr P. R. M. Steele, Dr W. Taylor, Dr G. Terenghi, Dr K. S. Vasudev, Dr G. T. Williams and Professor E. A. Wright. I would like to thank as well the secretaries Mrs Margery Clark, Mrs Alison Rawlinson and Miss Collette Youd for their competent work on the typescript and Mrs Christine Jarvis and other members of the technical staff for much time spent on re-cutting and re-staining sections. I am particularly grateful to Mr Alan Williams for his skill in preparing the iceberg of photomicrographs, the tip of which appears in this volume. Mr Barry Shurlock and latterly Dr Peter Altman of Chapman and Hall showed remarkable forbearance during the prolonged gestational period of this book and offered much helpful advice and encouragement, for which I thank them sincerely.

1 Introduction

This chapter will consider those aspects concerned with the taking and handling of upper gastrointestinal tract biopsies which are essential prerequisites for accurate diagnosis. This is followed by a description of certain types of artefact which may be seen in histological sections of material from this site.

1.1 Instruments

Most examinations of the upper gastrointestinal tract are carried out with forward-viewing endoscopes, but in particular circumstances, e.g. lesions in the oesophagus and certain parts of the duodenum, a repeat examination with a lateral-viewing instrument may give a better view and the opportunity to take more satisfactory biopsies.

The major factor which determines the size of the tissue samples is the diameter of the biopsy channel of the endoscope (Fig. 1.1). Recent developments in endoscopy design have resulted in instruments with a larger biopsy channel diameter relative to their overall diameter. The type of forceps used also affects the size of the biopsies and ellipsoid cups produce larger specimens than round cups (Danesh *et al.*, 1985). Toothed or spiked forceps have been advocated in the oesophagus, which is the least satisfactory site in the upper gastrointestinal tract for biopsy, probably due to the tangential approach necessary with forward-viewing endoscopes and the nature of the epithelium, which is smoother and firmer than that of the stomach or small intestine. Further details concerning practical aspects of endoscopy may be found in standard textbooks (Demling *et al.*, 1982; Cotton and Williams, 1982).

1.2 Handling of biopsies

Formol-saline or neutral buffered formaldehyde is an adequate fixative for routine use. Other fixatives, such as chilled buffered glutaraldehyde

1

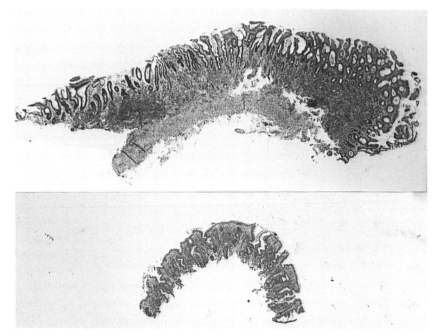

Fig. 1.1   Gastric biopsies removed using endoscopes with a 2 mm diameter (below) and a 3.7 mm diameter biopsy channel (above). HE × 22.5.

for ultrastructural studies and Bouin's solution for the examination of endocrine cells, are used in appropriate circumstances. Biopsies should be gently teased from the forceps into the fixative solution with a small needle. Shaking the end of the forceps in the fixative to dislodge the tissue may result in fragmentation, particularly in the case of duodenal samples.

In general, orientation of biopsies is unnecessary before they are placed in fixative. The samples are small, and attempts to handle them may result in traumatic artefact. During fixation they tend to curl up with their luminal aspect outwards and they can be optimally embedded for orientated sections to be cut. As well as this the number of biopsies taken in a single case (which may be 10 to 20 from a suspicious looking ulcer for example) makes it impracticable to individually orientate them. The important qualifications however are that the material should be handled by experienced technical staff, and that biopsies must be sectioned at different levels (see below), which nearly always results in adequately orientated material in the deeper cuts. Larger specimens, obtained for example with a suction capsule technique or via an endoscope with a wide diameter biopsy channel, can benefit from orientation, when samples are carefully placed submucosal surface downwards on a ground-glass slide or on plastic or nylon mesh before slowly immersing in fixative. This applies for example to suction biopsy specimens from the oesophagus removed for the assessment of possible reflux changes or oesophagitis (Section 3.1.3), and to biopsies from the second part of the duodenum to diagnose or exclude coeliac disease (Section 11.2). In the latter situation however villous architecture can be satisfactorily determined, without pre-fixation orientation, if enough biopsies (a minimum of four) are taken (Fig. 1.2).

How exhaustively biopsies are examined histologically in routine diagnostic practice depends on the workload of the individual pathologist. However it is essential that more than one level is looked at, since changes such as inflammation and neoplasia are frequently focal. As well as this, scrutiny of different levels usually gives a more 'dynamic' appraisal of the appearances which are present. The examination of different levels also means that several tissue samples (up to a maximum of five or six) may be included in a single block, and any slight misalignment in the plane in which the individual pieces are embedded is

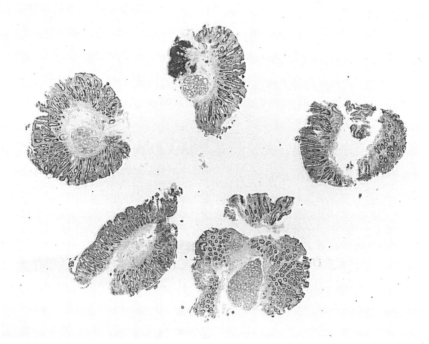

Fig. 1.2 In four of these five samples from the second part of the duodenum an adequate assessment of mucosal architecture (sub-total villous atrophy) is possible at this level. The biopsies were not orientated before being placed in fixative. HE × 13.5.

compensated for. I have found that examination of three levels of normal-sized biopsy samples, with three to four serial sections on each slide, is satisfactory. Two unstained spare sections, prepared at each level, ensure that special stains can be carried out when necessary. In addition, a routine periodic acid-Schiff/alcian blue stain at pH 2.5 on the middle level is particularly helpful in delineating areas of intestinal metaplasia in gastric biopsies and to detect small groups of mucin-containing carcinoma cells in the lamina propria (Fig. 9.12). Other situations where this stain is helpful include the demonstration of foci of gastric metaplasia in the superficial epithelium of the duodenum (Fig. 11.7), the assessment of the basal cell thickness of the oesophageal epithelium (apparent as negative staining compared to the superficial glycogen-containing PAS positive cells) and the staining of certain fungi, including *Candida* spp., which are PAS positive (Fig. 3.16).

1.3 Clinico-pathological liaison

Close co-operation and communication between pathologist and clinician is an essential part of biopsy interpretation and diagnosis. At one level this relates to information conveyed by the endoscopist to the pathologist on the request form accompanying biopsy specimens. This should include a brief clinical history, the endoscopic appearances and, most importantly, the site from which the tissue samples were taken. This is particularly necessary in the stomach in the evaluation of gastritis, where metaplasia of the body mucosa can result in an appearance indistinguishable from pyloric mucosa (Section 6.2.1(b)). It is also vital to know the levels at which biopsies are taken in order to diagnose a columnar-lined (Barrett's) oesophagus (Section 3.2). When multiple biopsies are taken from different sites this may be conveniently recorded on a rubber stamp organ outline.

Regular biopsy meetings between gastroenterologist and pathologist are extremely valuable. They allow demonstration of interesting case material, discussion of problem cases, and provide an important forum for teaching. In the same way occasional visits by the pathologist to the endoscopy suite are often informative and enable him (or her) to suggest improvements in the way the specimens are collected or handled.

1.4 Artefacts

Minor degrees of separation of foveolae and to a lesser extent of glands due to oedema are sometimes seen in biopsies from the stomach and duodenum which are otherwise normal. They are probably related to the endoscopic procedure. Distended capillaries and foci of extravasated red

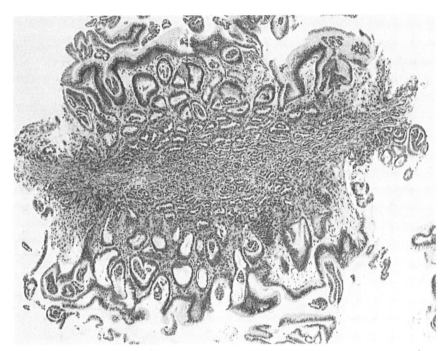

Fig. 1.3 A misleading appearance suggesting infiltrating carcinoma in this crushed and poorly orientated gastric biopsy. HE × 60.

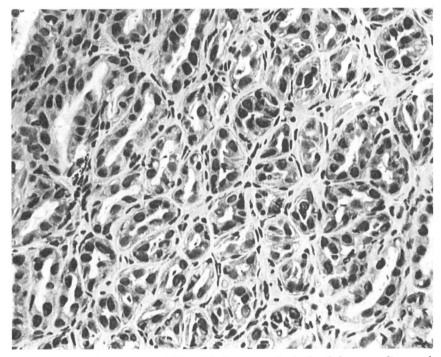

Fig. 1.4 A higher power of Fig. 1.3 shows marked glandular crowding and nuclear hyperchromatism. HE × 375.

blood cells may also be present and are more frequent and conspicuous in biopsies obtained by suction techniques.

A more common and potentially important change results from crushing of tissue by the biopsy forceps. Glandular crowding and hyperchromasia of nuclei may in particular circumstances give a superficial resemblance to carcinoma (Figs 1.3 and 1.4). The site where the piece of tissue has been pinched or grasped is however usually obvious. Lymphoid infiltrates, both benign and malignant, often show considerable crush artefact which can make interpretation difficult in material where they are a prominent component. Crushing of Brunner's glands in duodenal biopsies is frequent and results in a fibrillary appearance of the mucin which on occasion may give rise to a slightly confusing appearance when these glands have extended into the mucosa (Fig. 1.5). Another common

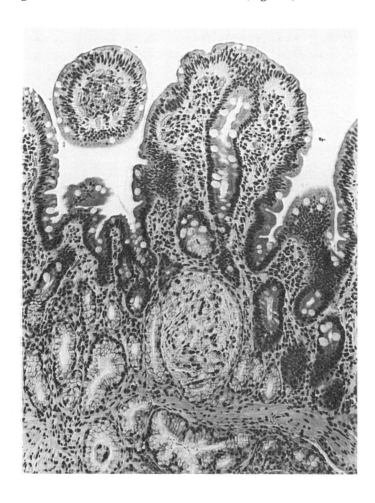

effect of compression is seen in biopsies from the gastric body and to a lesser extent in samples from other sites in the stomach. In the former case, groups of well-preserved parietal, chief and mucous cells are present lying in the lumen of the upper glands or pits (Fig. 1.6). This change occurs in both normal and inflamed gastric mucosa and is not present in sections from resection specimens, so that it is not a result of increased cell turnover as some observers have suggested.

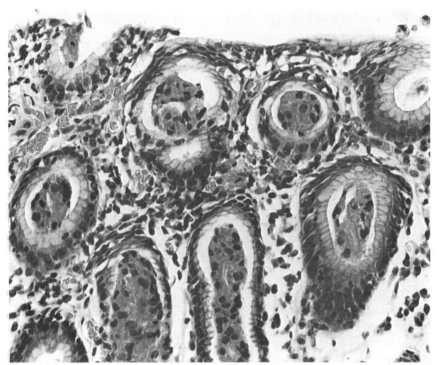

Fig. 1.6   Groups of body cells in the gastric pits with some flattening of the surface epithelium. HE × 292.

Extraneous material which may accompany tissue samples includes pieces of food and barium. The former is most likely in situations where there are obstructing or stenotic lesions. Sometimes food particles become sequestered in the floor of a deep ulcer. The type of barium sulphate commonly used in double-contrast radiological examinations of the upper gastrointestinal tract consists of crushed high density preparations and is apparent in histological sections as large (up to 50 μm

Fig. 1.5   Crush artefact affecting a Brunner's gland in the duodenal mucosa. HE × 135.

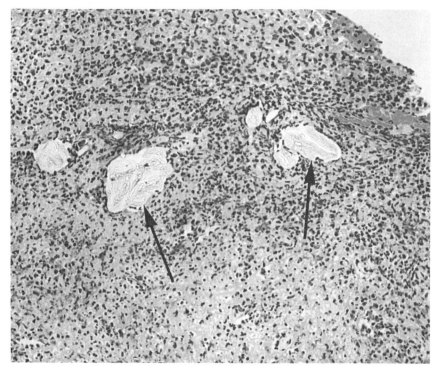

Fig. 1.7 Barium sulphate crystals (arrowed) embedded in granulation tissue from an oesophageal ulcer. HE × 190.

maximum dimension), bi-refringent, rhomboidal crystals which are incorporated into granulation tissue (Fig. 1.7) or coat the slough of ulcers and erosions (Levison *et al.*, 1984; Womack, 1984).

References

Cotton, P.B. and Williams, C.B. (1982), *Practical Gastrointestinal Endoscopy*, Blackwell Scientific Publications, Oxford.

Danesh, B.J.Z., Burke, M., Newman, J. *et al.* (1985), Comparison of weight, depth and diagnostic adequacy of specimens obtained with 16 different biopsy forceps designed for upper gastrointestinal endoscopy. *Gut*, **26**, 227–231.

Demling, L., Elster, K., Koch, H. and Rosch, W. (1982), *Endoscopy and Biopsy of Esophagus, Stomach and Duodenum. A Colour Atlas*, W.B. Saunders, Philadelphia.

Levison, D.A., Crocker, P.R., Smith, A. *et al.* (1984), Varied light and scanning electron microscopic appearances of barium sulphate in smears and histological sections. *J. Clin. Pathol.*, **37**, 481–487.

Womack, C. (1984), Unusual histological appearances of barium sulphate – a case report with scanning electron microscopy and energy dispersive X-ray analysis. *J. Clin. Pathol.*, **37**, 488–493.

2 The normal oesophageal mucosa

2.1 Endoscopic appearances

In an adult the distance from the incisor teeth to the upper end of the oesophagus at the crico-pharyngeal sphincter is about 15 cm, and to the squamo-columnar junction about 40 cm. The latter is recognized as a serrated line (ora serrata, Z-line) with four to six long or short extensions, with the pink-coloured columnar epithelium standing slightly proud of the paler, smooth and shiny squamous epithelium. The meeting of these epithelia does not coincide with the anatomical gastro-oesophageal junction but occurs a short distance proximally at about diaphragmatic level and in the distal part of the lower oesophageal sphincter, a 3–5 cm long high pressure zone at the lower end of the oesophagus. It follows therefore that the oesophagus is lined by squamous epithelium except for a small segment at its lower end which consists of surface mucin-secreting columnar epithelium with underlying mucous glands. This continues a short but variable distance into the stomach where it is usually referred to as cardiac mucosa. Since it is common to both sites the term junctional mucosa has been proposed (Hayward, 1961).

2.2 Histology

2.2.1 *Squamous-lined mucosa*

This is some 500–800 µm thick and is composed of non-keratinizing stratified squamous epithelium with underlying lamina propria and muscularis mucosae (Fig. 2.1). The squamous epithelium has a basal zone consisting of several layers of cuboidal or oblong basophilic cells with dark nuclei in which glycogen is absent. It occupies some 10–15% of the thickness of the normal epithelium although it may be increased in the last 2 cm or so of the squamous-lined oesophagus (Section 3.1.3). Occasional mitoses are seen in the basal cell layer. Above the basal zone

9

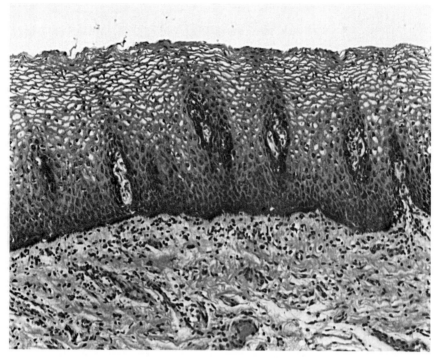

Fig. 2.1   Normal oesophageal squamous epithelium with narrow basal zone and papillae extending just over half way into its total thickness. HE × 114.

the epithelial cells are larger and become progressively flattened, but even on the surface retain their nuclei. Keratohyalin granules are not present in the surface cells of normal epithelium. Glycogen is abundant. Single intraepithelial lymphocytes lying between the squamous cells are common, particularly in the lower half of the mucosa.

Both melanocytes and non-melanocyte argyrophil cells can occur randomly distributed in the basal layer of the epithelium, the former usually as small groups and the latter singly (De la Pava *et al.*, 1963; Tateishi *et al.*, 1974). They are presumably the source of the rare primary malignant melanomas and oat cell carcinomas that occur at this site.

The lower border of the epithelium is irregular due to the presence of numerous conical vascular papillae of connective tissue which project upwards from the lamina propria to reach as far as two-thirds of the way into the total thickness of the epithelium. The lamina propria consists of loose connective tissue in which there are a sprinkling of lymphocytes, plasma cells and an occasional eosinophil and mast cell. Focal collections of lymphocytes and plasma cells may be aggregated around the ducts of the submucosal glands (Fig. 2.2).

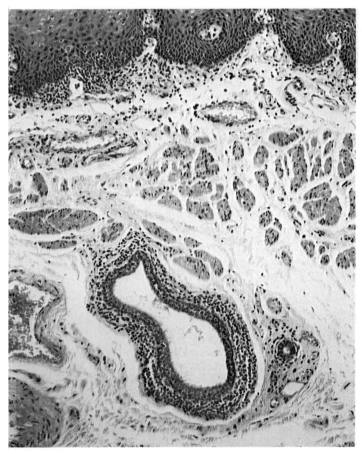

Fig. 2.2 Collection of lymphocytes surround the duct of a submucosal oesophageal gland. HE × 129.

The muscularis mucosae in the upper part of the oesophagus is less well developed than lower down where it consists of a continuous sheet of longitudinal and transverse fibres and may reach up to 300 μm in thickness at the squamo-columnar junction.

2.2.2 Junctional mucosa

At the lower end of the oesophagus there is a sudden change from stratified squamous epithelium to mucin-secreting columnar epithelium which dips down at intervals to form pits or foveolae, into which compound or branched tubular glands open (Fig. 2.3). At the upper end of this zone, groups of these glands which branch freely and pursue a

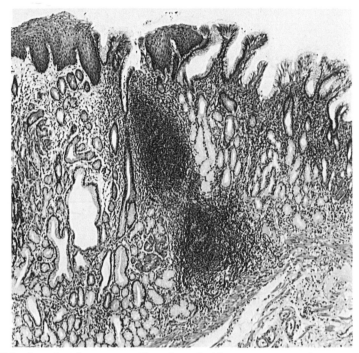

Fig. 2.3 Junctional mucosa. Note lymphoid aggregates and cystic glands. HE × 60.

tortuous course, are aggregated into lobules by thin septa of collagen and fibres derived from the muscularis mucosae (Fig. 2.4). This lobular arrangement disappears distally, with glands becoming less branched, and here the mucosa is thinner. The transition from this zone to the fundic glands is gradual. The junctional glands often extend a short distance deep to the oesophageal squamous epithelium (Fig. 2.5) or occur in small groups just above the squamo-columnar junction, and in this situation have been referred to as superficial glands of the oesophagus (see below). The extension of the junctional mucosa distally varies considerably, usually being of the order of 0.5–1.5 cm but can be as much as 3–4 cm.

The majority of the gland cells are mucous and stain strongly with the PAS method. Occasional cells near the upper end of the glands close to the squamous junction may secrete both sialo- and sulphomucins (Gad, 1969). Parietal cells, morphologically identical to those in the fundic glands, are present in small numbers, and occasionally chief cells as well. Numerous endocrine cells, some of which are argentaffin and others argyrophil, are found in this region (Krause *et al.*, 1978).

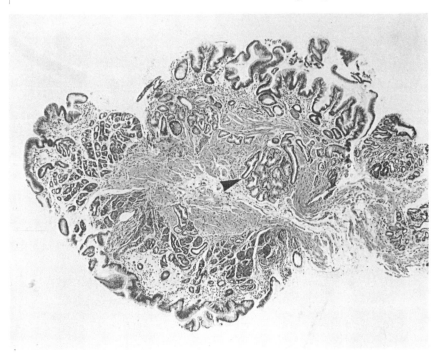

Fig. 2.4 Junctional mucosa. Lobulate appearance of mucous glands with sur-rounding smooth muscle fibres (arrowed) in this biopsy from below the squamo-columnar junction. HE × 38.

Cystic change is common particularly near the squamous junction and can occur close to the opening of the glands into the foveolae or deeper (Fig. 2.3). Lymphoid follicles are also common in the deeper part of the mucosa or extending through the muscularis mucosae into the submucosa.

2.2.3 Superficial glands of the oesophagus

As well as occurring at the lower end of the oesophagus (see above), small islands of glandular mucosa are not uncommon at post-mortem on the lateral walls of the oesophagus from the level of the cricoid to that of the fifth tracheal cartilage (Hewlett, 1901; Taylor, 1927). These areas may be mistaken at endoscopy for erosions or small ulcers and biopsied. Like junctional mucosa they consist of branching tubular glands, which may show cystic dilatation, lined by mucous cells and a few parietal cells.

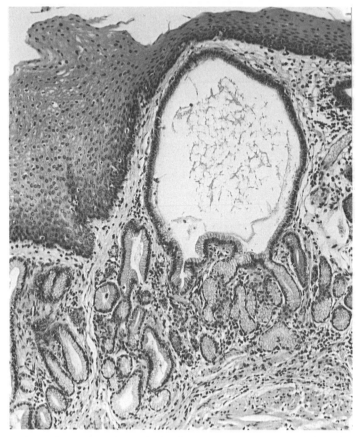

Fig. 2.5 Superficial oesophageal glands. Mucous glands with focal dilatation beneath squamous epithelium. HE × 115.

2.2.4 Deep glands of the oesophagus

These tubulo-alveolar glands, which contain sulphomucins, are submucosal (Fig. 2.6) and therefore rarely seen in biopsy material although their ducts may be present. These are lined by stratified squamous epithelium and surrounded by lymphocytes and plasma cells.

2.2.5 Ciliated epithelium in the oesophagus

This appears normally in the foetus at the 40 mm stage as a superficial layer of the stratified columnar epithelium and becomes replaced by stratified squamous epithelium at approximately the 130 mm stage, beginning in the middle third of the oesophagus (Johns, 1952). Small

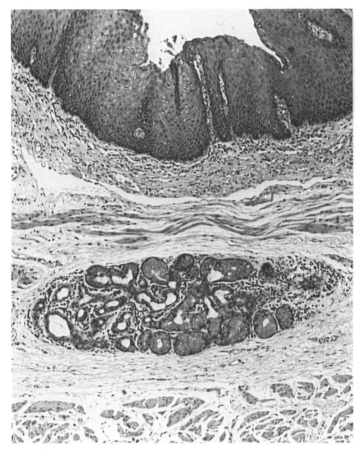

Fig. 2.6   Submucosal oesophageal gland. HE × 77.

islands of ciliated epithelium may be present at birth however, but appear to be rapidly desquamated (Rector and Connerley, 1941). There is one case report of similar epithelium found in the lower half of the oesophagus at post-mortem in an adult (Raeburn, 1951).

References

De la Pava, S., Nigogosyan, G., Pickren, J.W. and Cabrera, A. (1963), Melanosis of the esophagus. *Cancer*, **16**, 48–50.

Gad, A. (1969), A histochemical study of human alimentary tract mucosubstances in health and disease. I. Normal and tumours. *Br. J. Cancer*, **23**, 52–63.

Hayward, J. (1961), The lower end of the oesophagus. *Thorax*, **16**, 36–41.

Hewlett, A.W. (1901), The superficial glands of the oesophagus. *J. Exp. Med.*, **5**, 319–331.

Johns, B.A.E. (1952), Developmental changes in the oesophageal epithelium in man. *J.Anat.*, **86**, 431–442.

Krause, W.J., Ivey, K.J., Baskin, W.N. and MacKercher, P.A. (1978), Morphological observations on the normal human cardiac glands. *Anat. Rec.*, **192**, 59–72.

Raeburn, C. (1951), Columnar ciliated epithelium in the adult oesophagus. *J. Pathol. Bacteriol.*, **63**, 157–158.

Rector, L.E. and Connerley, M.L. (1941), Aberrant mucosa in the esophagus in infants and in children. *Arch. Pathol.*, **31**, 285–294.

Tateishi, R., Taniguchi, H., Wada, A. *et al.* (1974), Argyrophil cells and melanocytes in esophageal mucosa. *Arch. Pathol.*, **98**, 87–89.

Taylor, A.L. (1927), The epithelial heterotopias of the alimentary tract. *J. Pathol. Bacteriol.*, **30**, 415–449.

3 Oesophagitis

Inflammation of the oesophagus is most often due to a reflux of material from the stomach, but can occur with various types of infection, after the ingestion of noxious material, or following irradiation. It is frequently present in the mucosa adjacent to tumours. The oesophagus may rarely be affected in Crohn's disease or in eosinophilic gastroenteritis and oeosophageal involvement can be a feature of several skin disorders. A desquamative oesophagitis with web formation affecting the upper and mid-oesophagus has been described in patients with chronic graft-versus-host disease following allogeneic bone marrow transplantation (McDonald *et al.*, 1981).

3.1 Reflux oesophagitis

3.1.1 Pathogenesis

Some degree of gastro-oesophageal reflux is commonplace, occurring for example in healthy individuals after meals (Kaye, 1977), and during early pregnancy (Fisher *et al.*, 1978). When excessive, however, inflammation of the lower oesophagus results and this may be accompanied by erosions and ulceration. Extension of the inflammation deep into the wall with associated fibrosis can result in a stricture. In some cases of reflux oesophagitis the stratified squamous epithelium is replaced by columnar epithelium, so-called Barrett's oesophagus. This is discussed below (Section 3.2).

Gastro-oesophageal reflux disease occurs in many clinical settings and its pathogenesis is almost certainly multifactorial (Dodds *et al.*, 1981). A sliding hiatus hernia is a common, although not essential accompaniment and sometimes there is an associated duodenal ulcer (Goldman *et al.*, 1967). It may follow nasogastric intubation, repeated vomiting, operations which interfere with the gastro-oesophageal junction, and surgical vagotomy. It can also occur in alcoholic and diabetic autonomic neuropathy and in scleroderma. Persistent or transient loss of tone of the lower oesophageal sphincter is generally accepted as the major determinant of the reflux although interference with non-sphincteric anatomical mechanisms is probably also important. Delay in emptying of the stomach (Baldi *et al.*, 1981; McCallum *et al.*, 1981) and duodeno-gastric regurgitation (Gillison *et al.*, 1969; Kaye and Showalter, 1974) have been present in some patients and indicate the need to consider a more generalized abnormality of the upper gastrointestinal tract in the causation of this disorder. Whether or not inflammation or reflux changes (see below) result probably depends on a number of factors including the volume and nature of the refluxate, the efficiency of secondary peristalsis in clearing the oesophagus of refluxed material, the resistance of the oesophageal epithelium to injury, and the neutralizing effects of bicarbonate rich saliva and secretions from the oesophageal glands.

3.1.2 Endoscopic appearances

The earliest changes are diffuse or patchy hyperaemia or erythema of the distal oesophageal mucosa which on close inspection is due to a marked widening and irregularity of small blood vessels, present in the normal mucosa as fine parallel longitudinal red lines (Hattori *et al.*, 1974). The normally clear demarcation of squamous and columnar epithelium may become indistinct or effaced. At a more advanced stage the mucosa is friable and bleeds easily when touched. Linear erosions, surrounded by a red halo and covered by a yellow exudate which can be wiped off, occur first on the longitudinal folds of the posterior wall of the oesophagus some 1–2 cm proximal to the Z-line. With increasing severity, erosions are multiple, confluent and may eventually involve the whole circumference of the lower oesophagus. Features of chronic disease include a nodular appearance of the mucosa, poor distensibility of the oesophageal wall, the presence of a stricture, and ulceration. Single or multiple inflammatory polyps can occur (Rabin *et al.*, 1980). Fibrous septum formation resulting in a double lumen (Mihas *et al.*, 1976) and multiple oesophago-gastric fistulae (Raymond *et al.*, 1980) have also been reported as complications of long-standing disease.

In the majority of cases the appearances at endoscopy, particularly when there is erosive or ulcerative disease, correlate with histological evidence of inflammation in targeted biopsies. Patients with minor or equivocal features, or those with a normal appearance but who have symptoms of reflux or who have reflux on clinical investigation, may show little or no evidence of inflammation on histological examination but instead a number of features which have been designated as reflux changes (Ismail-Biegi *et al.*, 1970).

3.1.3 Histology

(a) *Reflux changes.* These consist of basal cell hyperplasia, so that this zone makes up more than 15% of the total thickness of the oesophageal epithelium, and extension of the papillae more than two-thirds of the distance to the surface (Fig. 3.1). These changes have been found randomly distributed over the distal 8 cm of the oesophagus (Ismail-Beigi and Pope, 1974). It is presumed that the basal zone thickening occurs as a result of an increased cellular proliferation in response to chronic low-grade oesophageal injury, and *in vitro* studies have shown a high labelling index in the basal zone of squamous mucosa with marked changes compared with normal controls (Livstone *et al.*, 1977).

It is generally agreed, however, that these appearances can occur normally in the lowermost 2 cm of the squamous-lined oesophageal mucosa as a result of 'physiological' reflux, and even with biopsies from higher levels some observers have found a poor correlation between the

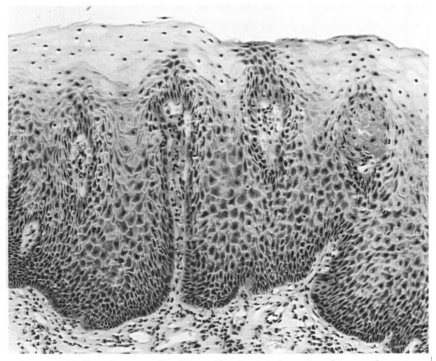

Fig. 3.1 Reflux changes. In this well-orientated suction biopsy there is an increase of the basal zone to occupy some 50% of the thickness of the epithelium, together with elongation of the dermal papillae which approach close to the surface. HE × 150.

changes and the demonstration of reflux (Weinstein *et al.*, 1975; Seefeld *et al.*, 1977; Adami *et al.*, 1979). As well as this these, histological features have been described in suction biopsies which contain underlying lamina propria and often muscularis mucosae as well as epithelium, and because of their size can be easily orientated. Biopsies taken with fibre-optic instruments from intact oesophageal mucosa are small, thus precluding orientation, with less than half the specimens containing lamina propria. In such material the presence of overlapping capillaries seen on tangentially cut specimens (Fig. 3.2) has been suggested as indicative of reflux (Kobayashi and Kasugai, 1974), as has the finding of markedly dilated capillaries high up in the epithelium surrounded by flattened epithelial cells containing pyknotic nuclei and sometimes associated with the

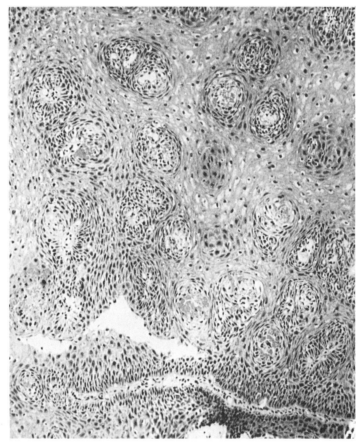

Fig. 3.2 Overlapping capillaries seen on this tangentially cut biopsy have been proposed as a criterion indicating reflux changes. HE × 132.

extravasation of red blood cells (Geboes *et al.*, 1980). In a study of children with acid reflux (Winter *et al.*, 1982) the presence of even occasional eosinophils in the oesophageal epithelium appeared to be a specific and earlier marker of peptic injury than other features such as basal zone hyperplasia and papillary length. These observations await confirmation in adults.

In summary, reflux changes reflect an increased cell turnover of the oesophageal epithelium which in the lowermost oesophagus is probably physiological but if present 2 cm or more above the squamo-columnar junction is abnormal. The changes are optimally assessed in orientated suction biopsies which include the whole thickness of the mucosa. In material obtained with a fibre-optic instrument the recognition of reflux changes is more difficult. In practice the important distinction is from oesophagitis where damage to the mucosa may lead to complications such as bleeding and stricture formation. Small biopsies obtained with flexible instruments should be step-sectioned and multiple biopsies taken when symptoms and/or endoscopic appearances dictate.

(b) *Oesophagitis*. Milder forms of oesophagitis are recognized in endo-scopic biopsies by the presence of small numbers of polymorphs in the lamina propria and infiltrating the squamous epithelium. There may be accompanying reflux changes. With more severe inflammation there are increased numbers of acute inflammatory cells often associated with oedema (Figs 3.3 and 3.4), manifest in the epithelium as widening of the intercellular spaces. Lamellar detachment may follow so that eventually only a thin layer of squamous epithelium is present overlying an acutely inflamed lamina propria in which capillary proliferation is prominent and in which there are increased numbers of lymphocytes and plasma cells (Fig. 3.5). Necrotic slough, granulation and fibrous tissue are prominent components of biopsies from strictures and ulcers (Fig. 3.6) and these should always be step-sectioned in a search for malignancy.

3.2   Columnar-lined (Barrett's) oesophagus

In some individuals with reflux oesophagitis, and for reasons which are not clear, the stratified squamous epithelium is replaced by columnar epithelium. This change is more common in males than females and has been identified in 0.5–4% of upper gastrointestinal endoscopic examina-tions (Savary and Miller, 1978; Burbige and Radigan, 1979; Stadelmann *et al.*, 1981). It occurs predominantly in later decades but is being increas-ingly recognized in children (Dahms and Rothstein, 1984). It was first described by Barrett (1950) who mistakenly considered it as a congenital short oesophagus with an attenuated intrathoracic stomach. It was

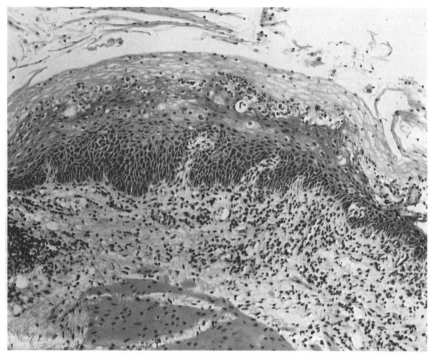

Fig. 3.3   Reflux oesophagitis. Infiltration of the epithelium and lamina propria by moderate numbers of polymorphs associated with incipient desquamation of the surface layers. HE × 105.

subsequently realized that the columnar epithelium present was lining the anatomical oesophagus (Allison and Johnstone, 1953; Cohen *et al.*, 1963) and because of the common association of the condition with a history and radiological evidence of gastro-oesophageal reflux is generally considered to be an acquired disorder in which progressive replacement of the squamous epithelium by columnar epithelium at the lower end of the oesophagus occurs (Goldman and Beckman, 1960; Mossberg, 1966; Endo *et al.*, 1974). A columnar-lined oesophagus has been described in patients with scleroderma and treated achalasia (Cameron and Payne, 1978; Berges *et al.*, 1980), and has also developed following partial oesophago-gastrectomy with anastomosis between squamous-lined oesophagus and gastric fundus (Hamilton and Yardley, 1977), after total gastrectomy with oesophago-jejunal anastomosis (Meyer *et al.*, 1979), and, as a localized change, at the site of a lye stricture (Spechler *et al.*, 1981).

Oral extension of gastric epithelium to replace damaged squamous epithelium obviously cannot satisfactorily explain the development of a

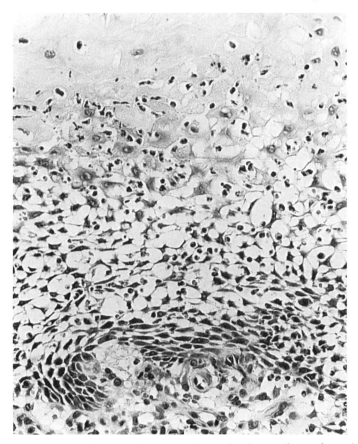

Fig. 3.4   Reflux oesophagitis. Large numbers of polymorphs in the epithelium with prominent intercellular oedema. HE × 262.

columnar-lined oesophagus in all these situations and alternative mechanisms could be by metaplasia of stratified squamous epithelium or hyperplasia of superficial oesophageal glands. It is also possible that some cases may be congenital (Stadelmann *et al.*, 1981), although this is generally considered unlikely.

There are conflicting reports as to whether or not columnar mucosa may regress following a successful anti-reflux operation (Naef *et al.*, 1975; Brand *et al.*, 1980; Hamilton *et al.*, 1984) or with non-operative treatment (Wesdorp *et al.*, 1981; Patel *et al.*, 1982). This is an important question to answer because Barrett's oesophagus is a premalignant condition, as increasing numbers of reports of dysplasia and carcinoma in such patients testify (Naef *et al.*, 1975; McDonald *et al.*, 1977; Berenson *et al.*, 1978; Haggitt *et al.*, 1978; Witt *et al.*, 1983). The prevalence of malignant

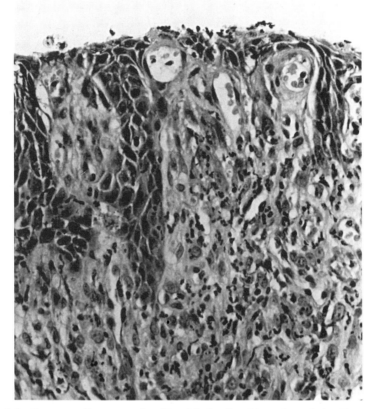

Fig. 3.5 Severe reflux oesophagitis. Markedly thinned and focally eroded epithelium overlies actively inflamed granulation tissue. HE × 322.

change is not known nor whether possible risk factors such as length of history or the extent of the change in the oesophagus are important in its development. In the present state of knowledge it would appear advisable that this group of patients are regularly endoscoped, when multiple biopsies and cytology can be carried out.

3.2.1 Endoscopic appearances

The endoscopic appearances in Barrett's oesophagus are of a velvety, orange-red mucosa lining the lower oesophagus and extending a variable distance proximally. The wall of the oesophagus is hypotonic and no longitudinal folds are present. This mucosa is often seen below a high peptic stricture accompanied by varying degrees of oesophagitis. A deep,

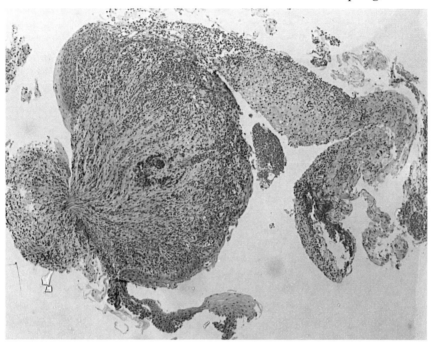

Fig. 3.6 Ulcer slough and granulation tissue are the predominant components of this biopsy from an oesophageal stricture secondary to reflux oesophagitis. HE × 60.

punched-out peptic ulcer may be present either at the junction of the columnar and squamous mucosa (Wolf *et al.*, 1955) or within the segment of columnar-lined oesophagus, so-called Barrett's ulcer (Barrett, 1950). A small hiatus hernia is common. The lower oesophagus may be completely lined by columnar mucosa or there may be residual islands of squamous mucosa and these have been identified at endoscopy by instillation of Lugol's solution, where they stain black in contrast to the unstained columnar mucosa (Burbige and Radigan, 1979). Dysplastic changes can occur in a flat mucosa or result in a nodular or polypoid appearance of the affected oesophagus.

3.2.2 Histology

Biopsies from columnar-lined oesophagus show a heterogeneous morphology regarding both gland type and surface architecture and often seen in material from the same individual (Paull *et al.*, 1976; Thompson *et al.*, 1983). The most common variety is epithelium with a flat or villiform surface composed of a mixture of columnar cells and intestinal-type goblet cells, with underlying crypt-like glands in which the same cell types, together with endocrine cells, are present (Figs 3.7 and 3.8).

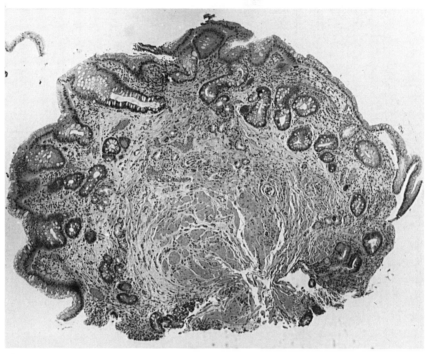

Fig. 3.7 Columnar-lined oesophagus. Biopsy taken at 28 cm shows a flat and atrophic mucosa with minor patchy inflammation. HE × 48.

Uncommonly, Paneth cells are seen at the base of the glands. The columnar cells, also known as intermediate (Jass, 1981) or principal (Trier, 1970) cells, have a variably developed brush border and contain apical mucin in their cytoplasm i.e. they have characteristics of both absorptive and secretory cells. Other types of mucosa present are an atrophic gastric fundal type with parietal and chief cells which tends to occur distally in the columnar-lined oesophagus, and cardiac type or junctional mucosa similar to that found at the normal squamo-columnar junction. All these appearances are consistent however with an upward spread of cardiac (junctional) type mucosa in which there is complete or, much more often, incomplete intestinal metaplasia. Indeed similar changes are common in this type of mucosa when the squamo-columnar junction is not mis-

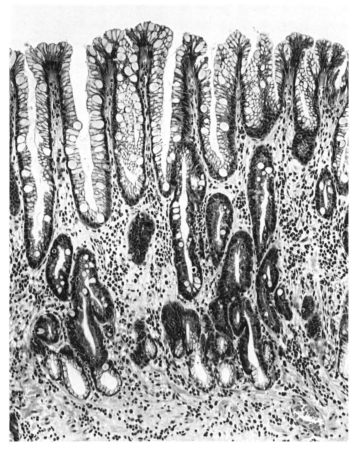

Fig. 3.8 Columnar-lined oesophagus. A villous pattern is present with surface epithelium composed of a mixture of goblet and intermediate cells. Similar cells line the glands except at the base where mucous cells containing neutral mucin are present. HE × 120.

placed. It follows from this therefore that it is essential to know both the endoscopic and radiological appearances and the level from which biopsies have been taken in order to diagnose a columnar-lined oesophagus. Occasionally the duct of an oesophageal sub-mucosal gland may be identified in a biopsy, and this is presumptive evidence that the material has been taken from the oesophagus (Fig. 3.9).

Active inflammation is common and regenerative changes may be conspicuous particularly with material removed from an ulcer edge. Biopsies from a high oesophageal stricture usually show granulation

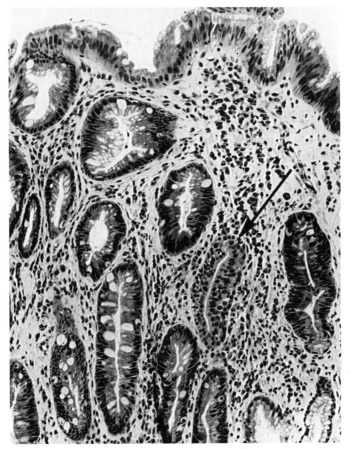

Fig. 3.9 Columnar-lined oesophagus. The duct of an oesophageal gland (arrowed) in the mucosa. HE × 150.

tissue and necrotic ulcer slough together with fragments of squamous or columnar mucosa (Fig. 3.10). Regenerative changes have to be distinguished from dysplasia and, as elsewhere in the gastrointestinal tract, this is not always straightforward. The recognition of dysplasia is facilitated in material which includes non-dysplastic mucosa as well. In obviously dysplastic epithelium cytological and architectural abnormalities are marked (Figs 3.11 and 3.12). Nuclei are enlarged, hyperchromatic and pleomorphic and there may be loss of polarity. Mitoses are often seen on the surface or in the upper parts of glands. There is a depletion of mucin. Glands may show dysplastic epithelium throughout their length or this change may be confined to their superficial portion (Fig. 3.13). The

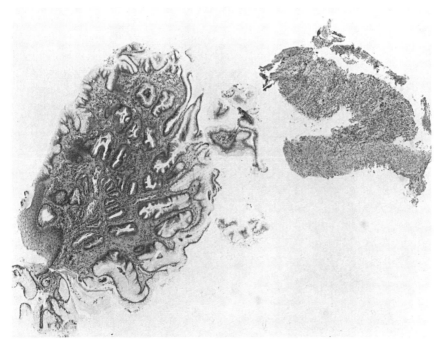

Fig. 3.10   Columnar-lined oesophagus. Inflamed squamo-columnar mucosa and ulcer slough in biopsies from a high oesophageal stricture. HE × 35.

surface may have a prominent papillary or villous configuration and in severe degrees of dysplasia there can be a back to back arrangement of glands. As in the stomach, distinction of severe dysplasia from intra-mucosal carcinoma may not be possible in biopsy material (Fig. 3.14). However, definite evidence of malignancy may be obvious and a similar range of histological appearances is seen as with gastric cancer. The finding of dysplasia in biopsy material is an indication for re-endoscopy with cytology and multiple biopsies.

3.3   Infective oesophagitis

Oesophagitis may occur in the course of such infectious diseases as measles, scarlet fever, diphtheria, smallpox and typhoid. In practice however specific infections which may be detected in oesophageal biopsy material are those caused by Candida, herpes simplex virus and cytome-galovirus, and tuberculosis. With the increasing use of immunosuppres-sive agents the first three of these in particular are occurring more

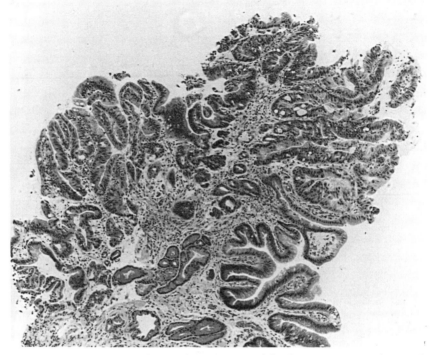

Fig. 3.11 Columnar-lined oesophagus. Most of this biopsy consists of severely dysplastic epithelium. HE × 59.

frequently, and accurate diagnosis is dependent on histology and culture of the organism involved.

3.3.1 Monilial oesophagitis

This is the commonest infective cause of oesophagitis and the causal agent is usually the dimorphic fungus *Candida albicans* although other organisms such as *Candida krusei* and *Torulopsis glabrata* (Jensen *et al.*, 1964) have also been isolated. *C. albicans* is normally a saprophyte but may become pathogenic under a variety of circumstances. Many of the reported cases have occurred in people with underlying malignancy, particularly myeloproliferative disorders (Eras *et al.*, 1972), in diabetics, following corticosteroid therapy or immunosuppressive drugs, or after the use of broad-spectrum antibiotics causing an alteration of the microecology of the gut flora. Some patients have had neutropenia (Holt, 1968). There may be accompanying oral thrush. At endoscopy, white patches or plaques are seen in the lower third of the oesophagus and may become confluent to form a pseudomembrane. Occasionally lesions may be

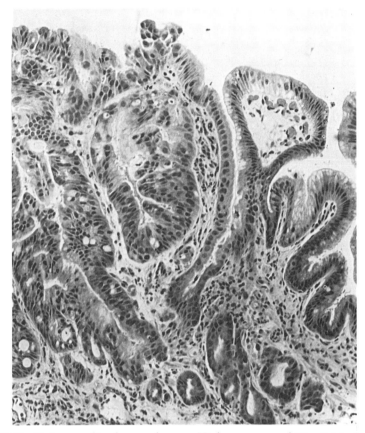

Fig. 3.12 Columnar-lined oesophagus. Higher power of Fig. 3.11 showing junction of non-dysplastic mucosa (right) with dysplastic area in which there is marked cytological and architectural atypia. HE × 150.

exophytic forming pseudotumours, and in chronic infections a cobble-stone appearance can result. In biopsy material the organism is seen as a pseudomycelium of non-branching hyphae some 2–3 μm in diameter, and as oval spores up to 4 μm in largest diameter, associated with ulcer slough or granulation tissue (Figs 3.15 and 3.16). If numerous they can be readily seen in routinely stained sections but when scanty their recognition is facilitated by a PAS, Grocott, or Gomori preparation. Brushing of suspicious lesions at endoscopy followed by direct smears has resulted in a higher detection rate than examination of histological material, and has correlated with high serum agglutinin titres (Kodsi *et al.*, 1976). Associated lesions in the upper gastrointestinal tract such as peptic ulcers and tumours of the oesophagus and stomach have been frequent (Kodsi *et al.*, 1976; Scott and Jenkins, 1982).

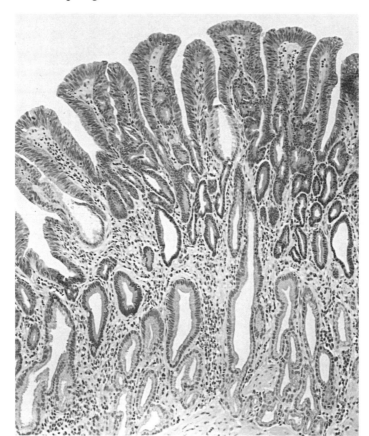

Fig. 3.13   Columnar-lined oesophagus. Minor to moderate dysplasia affecting the surface villous epithelium and upper parts of glands. HE × 111.

3.3.2 *Herpetic oesophagitis*

Although rarely suspected or diagnosed during life (McKay and Day, 1983) herpes simplex oesophagitis is not infrequently found at postmortem (Nash and Ross, 1974). The disease most frequently affects immunosuppressed patients with malignant disease, particularly malignant lymphomas and leukaemias, but may occur in a wide variety of clinical settings, e.g. following burns or after renal transplantation. A few cases have been reported of self-limited disease occurring in healthy adults (Owensby and Stammer, 1978; Springer *et al.*, 1979). The finding of small discrete vesicles with an erythematous base at endoscopy is fairly characteristic but with advanced disease these superficial lesions become

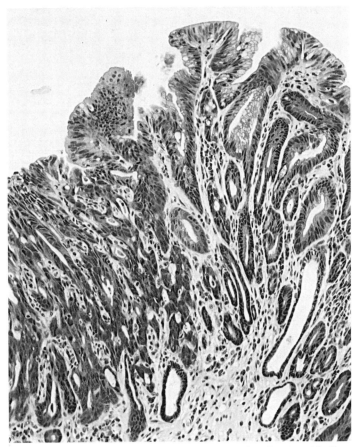

Fig. 3.14 Columnar-lined oesophagus. Moderately dysplastic epithelium on the right merges with an area showing glandular crowding, irregularity and budding. Whether these appearances represent severe dysplasia or intramucosal carcinoma is subjective. A subsequent resection specimen showed unequivocal invasive carcinoma. HE × 150.

confluent and the appearances non-specific. The lower third of the oesophagus is the site most commonly involved. Histologically there is partial or full thickness loss of the epithelium and infected cells at the margins of erosions contain homogeneous, round or oval Cowdry type A intranuclear viral inclusions (Fig. 3.17). Affected cells may be multinucleated. In desquamated necrotic cells the inclusions are palely basophilic with clumping of chromatin just inside the nuclear membrane (Fig. 3.18). Where the diagnosis is suspected the edges of ulcers should be biopsied to include infected epithelial cells. The ulcers can become

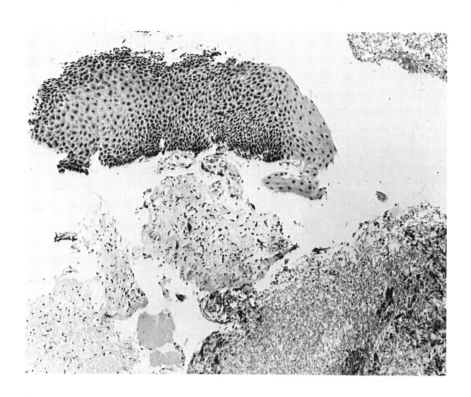

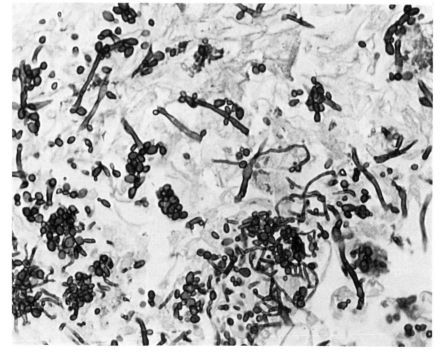

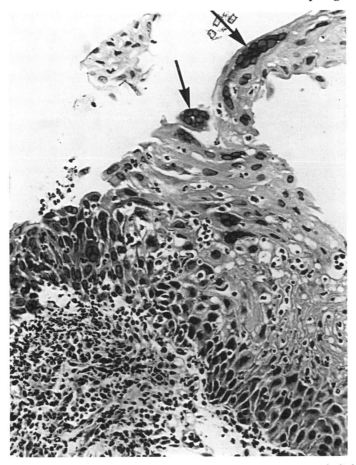

Fig. 3.17   Herpetic oesophagitis. Intranuclear viral inclusions in epithelial cells at left. Note multinucleated cells (arrowed). HE × 262.

secondarily infected particularly by Candida (Brayko *et al.*, 1982), and cytomegalovirus may also be seen in fibroblasts or endothelial cells of inflamed granulation tissue.

A giant oesophageal ulcer associated with cytomegalovirus inclusions and without evidence of invasive candidiasis has recently been described in a man with an acquired deficiency of cell-mediated immunity (Onge and Bezahler, 1982). The oesophagus may also be involved in patients with a thoracic distribution of herpes zoster (Gill *et al.*, 1984).

Fig. 3.15   Squamous epithelium, granulation tissue and fungal elements (bottom right). HE × 99.

Fig. 3.16   Hyphae and oval spores of *Candida albicans*. PAS/AB × 600.

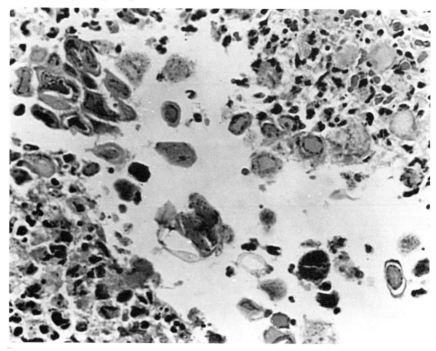

Fig. 3.18   Herpetic oesophagitis. Degenerate epithelial cells showing chromatin clumping around viral inclusions. HE × 600.

3.3.3 *Other infective agents*

Rarely tuberculosis (Weimann *et al.*, 1979; Dow, 1981) or histoplasmosis (Lee *et al.*, 1977; Schneider and Edwards, 1977) has manifested itself by oesophageal involvement, most commonly as a result of extension from affected mediastinal lymph nodes, and occasionally provided material at endoscopy from which a positive diagnosis could be made. A case has been reported of infection of the oesophagus caused by *Lactobacillus acidophilus* which endoscopically and radiologically was indistinguishable from moniliasis (McManus and Webb, 1975).

3.4   Other causes of oesophagitis

3.4.1 *Drugs*

A number of drugs swallowed as tablets or capsules have given rise to inflammation and ulceration of the oesophagus by a local irritative effect following hold-up (Kikendall *et al.*, 1983). Those most commonly implicated have been the anticholinergic agent emepronium bromide, doxycycline and tetracycline. The commonest site of damage has been the mid-oesophagus and the ulcers are discrete, often multiple, and may be serpiginous in outline. They usually heal without stricture formation. Most cases have been in people with a normal oesophagus where medication was taken with little or no fluid just before lying down. More severe cases, resulting in stricture formation, have occurred with slow-release potassium chloride tablets in patients with oesophageal obstruction (Collins *et al.*, 1979). The histological features in biopsies are non-specific and the diagnosis is a clinical one based on history and endoscopic findings.

3.4.2 Radiation-induced oesophagitis

Radiation therapy to the mediastinum may be followed by a self-limited but rarely severe oesophagitis. In some cases however serious complications such as ulcer, stricture and fistula formation can occur. Irradiation of squamous cell carcinomas of the oesophagus can result in a tracheo-oesophageal fistula and biopsies carried out to detect recurrent or residual carcinoma may show radiation changes with bizarre fibroblasts, oedema and an obliterative vasculitis (Figs 3.19 and 3.20). Serious effects, including stricture formation, may follow even low radiation doses when adjunctive chemotherapy with Adriamycin, daunorubicin or actinomycin D has been used (Greco *et al.*, 1976; Newburger *et al.*, 1978). Subsequent chemotherapy may result in recurrent oesophagitis.

3.4.3 Crohn's disease

Very rarely the oesophagus may be involved in patients with Crohn's disease affecting the small intestine or large bowel. Usually the lower part is affected and, depending on the stage of the disease, there is an erosive or ulcerative oesophagitis with or without stricture formation. Occasionally, characteristic endoscopic appearances may be visible with shallow and irregular aphthoid ulcers occurring in a normal mucosa (Huchzermeyer *et al.*, 1976), or there may be a cobblestone pattern, but more often the changes are non-specific. This often applies as well to the biopsy findings although non-caseating granulomas have occasionally been seen (Miller *et al.*, 1977).

Sarcoidosis affecting the gastrointestinal tract is uncommon but one biopsy confirmed case of oesophageal involvement is documented. (Polachek and Matre, 1964).

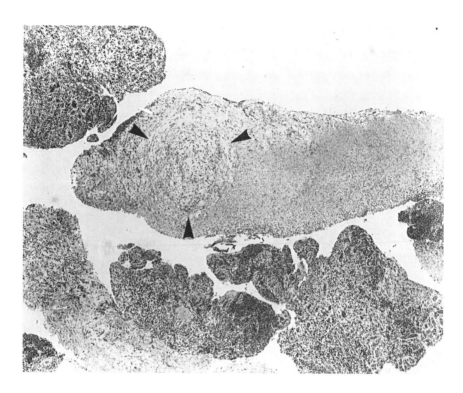

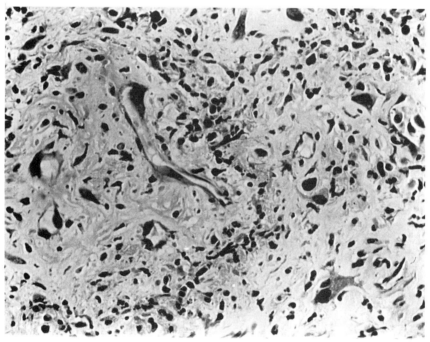

3.4.4 Eosinophilic oesophagitis

There are a few reports of oesophageal involvement in eosinophilic gastroenteritis (Dobbins *et al.*, 1977; Landres *et al.*, 1978). Some have been associated with motility disturbances such as diffuse spasm and achalasia. In biopsies there is elongation of the papillae, basal zone hyperplasia, and marked infiltration by eosinophils of the epithelium, lamina propria and muscularis mucosae (Fig. 3.21).

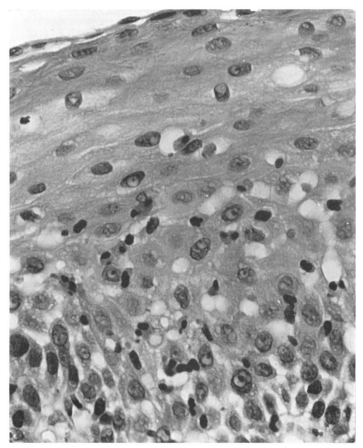

Fig. 3.21 Eosinophilic oesophagitis. Numerous eosinophils infiltrate squamous epithelium. HE × 600.

Fig. 3.19 Radiation oesophagitis. Granulation tissue and necrotic slough in oesophageal biopsies from patient with post-irradiation tracheo-oesophageal fistula. Obliterated arteriole is arrowed. HE × 38.

Fig. 3.20 Detail of Fig. 3.19 showing oedema, bizarre fibroblasts and swollen endothelial cells of capillaries. HE × 375.

3.4.5 Oesophagitis and skin diseases

Numerous skin diseases may involve the oesophagus including pemphigus vulgaris, bullous pemphigoid, benign mucosal pemphigoid, epidermolysis bullosa, toxic epidermal necrolysis (Lyell's disease), Stevens-Johnson syndrome, Darier's disease, tylosis palmaris et plantaris and acanthosis nigricans. The subject has been well reviewed (Geboes and Janssens, 1974). Multiple, discrete, shallow ulcers of the distal oesophagus separated by normal mucosa have been described in Behçet's syndrome (Lockhart *et al.*, 1976; Kaplinsky *et al.*, 1977). In systemic sclerosis absent peristalsis and loss of lower oesophageal sphincter tone predispose to reflux and oesophagitis (Atkinson and Summerling, 1966) and co-existent candidiasis is common (Cohen *et al.*, 1980). Columnar epithelium may line the lower oesophagus (Cameron and Payne, 1978).

References

Adami, B., Eckardt, V.F. and Paulini, K. (1979), Sampling error and observer variation in the interpretation of esophageal biopsies. *Digestion*, **19**, 404–410.

Allison, P.R. and Johnstone, A.S. (1953), The oesophagus lined with gastric mucous membrane. *Thorax*, **8**, 87–101.

Atkinson, M. and Summerling, M.D. (1966), Oesophageal changes in systemic sclerosis. *Gut*, **7**, 402–408.

Baldi, F., Corinaldesi, R., Ferrarini, F. *et al.* (1981), Gastric secretion and emptying of liquids in reflux esophagitis. *Dig. Dis. Sci.*, **26**, 886–889.

Barrett, N.R. (1950), Chronic peptic ulcer of the oesophagus and 'oesophagitis'. *Br. J. Surg.*, **38**, 175–182.

Berenson, M.M., Riddell, R.H., Skinner, D.B. and Freston, J.W. (1978), Malignant transformation of esophageal columnar epithelium. *Cancer*, **41**, 554–561.

Berges, W., Borchard, F., Strohmeyer, G. and Wienbeck, M. (1980), Columnar lined lower esophagus in primary motility disorders. *Gastroenterology*, **78**, 1140 (abstract).

Brand, D.L., Ylvisaker, J.T., Gelfand, M. and Pope, C.E. II (1980), Regression of columnar esophageal (Barrett's) epithelium after anti-reflux surgery. *N. Engl. J. Med.*, **302**, 844–848.

Brayko, C.M., Kozarek, R.A., Sanowski, R.A. and Lanard, B.J. (1982), Type I herpes simplex esophagitis with concomitant esophageal moniliasis. *J. Clin. Gastroenterol.*, **4**, 351–355.

Burbige, E.J. and Radigan, J.J. (1979), Characteristics of the columnar-cell lined (Barrett's) esophagus. *Gastrointest. Endosc.*, **25**, 133–136.

Cameron, A.J. and Payne, W.S. (1978), Barrett's esophagus occurring as a complication of scleroderma. *Mayo Clin. Proc.*, **53**, 612–615.

Cohen, B.R., Wolf, B.S., Som, M. and Janowitz, H.D. (1963), Correlation of manometric, oesophagoscopic, and radiological findings in the columnar-lined gullet (Barrett syndrome). *Gut*, **4**, 406–412.

Cohen, S., Laufer, I., Snape, W.J.Jr. *et al.*(1980), The gastrointestinal manifestations of scleroderma: pathogenesis and management. *Gastroenterology*, **79**, 155–166.

Collins, F.J., Mathews, H.R., Baker, S.E. and Strakova, J.M. (1979), Drug-induced oesophageal injury. *Br. Med. J.*, **i**, 1673–1676.

Dahms, B.B. and Rothstein, F.C. (1984), Barrett's esophagus in children: a consequence of chronic gastroesophageal reflux. *Gastroenterology*, **86**, 318–323.

Dobbins, J.W., Sheahan, D.G. and Behar, J. (1977), Eosinophilic gastroenteritis with esophageal involvement. *Gastroenterology*, **72**, 1312–1316.

Dodds, W.J., Hogan, W.J., Helm, J.F. and Dent, J. (1981), Pathogenesis of reflux esophagitis. *Gastroenterology*, **81**, 376–394.

Dow, C.J. (1981), Oesophageal tuberculosis: four cases. *Gut*, **22**, 234–236.

Endo, M., Kobayashi, S., Kozu, T. *et al.*(1974), A case of Barrett epithelization followed up for five years. *Endoscopy*, **6**, 48–51.

Eras, P., Goldstein, M.J. and Sherlock, P. (1972), Candida infection of the gastrointestinal tract. *Medicine (Baltimore)*, **51**, 367–379.

Fisher, R.S., Roberts, G.S., Grabowski, C.J. and Cohen, S. (1978), Altered lower esophageal sphincter function during early pregnancy. *Gastroenterology*, **74**, 1233–1237.

Geboes, K. and Janssens, J. (1974), The esophagus in cutaneous diseases. In *Diseases of the Esophagus* (ed. G.R. Vantrappen and J.J. Hellemans), Springer-Verlag, New York, Berlin, Heidelberg, pp. 823–833.

Geboes, K., Desmet, V., Vantrappen, G. and Mebis, J. (1980), Vascular changes in the esophageal mucosa. An early histologic sign of esophagitis. *Gastrointest. Endosc.*, **26**, 29–32.

Gill, R.A., Gebhard, R.L., Dozeman, R.L. and Sumner, H.W. (1984), Shingles esophagitis: endoscopic diagnosis in two patients. *Gastrointest. Endosc.*, **30**, 26–27.

Gillison, E.W., Capper, W.M., Airth, G.R. *et al.* (1969), Hiatus hernia and heartburn. *Gut*, **10**, 609–613.

Goldman, M.C. and Beckman, R.C. (1960), Barrett syndrome. Case report with discussion about concepts of pathogenesis. *Gastroenterology*, **39**, 104–110.

Goldman, M.S.Jr., Rasch, J.R., Wiltsie, D.S. and Finkel, M. (1967), The incidence of esophagitis in peptic ulcer disease. *Am. J. Dig. Dis.*, **12**, 994–999.

Greco, F.A., Brereton, H.D., Kent, H. *et al.* (1976), Adriamycin and enhanced radiation reaction in normal esophagus and skin. *Ann. Intern. Med.*, **85**, 294–298.

Haggitt, R.C., Tryzelaar, J., Ellis, F.H. and Colcher, H. (1978), Adenocarcinoma complicating columnar epithelium-lined (Barrett's) esophagus. *Am. J. Clin. Pathol.*, **70**, 1–5.

Hamilton, S.R. and Yardley, J.H. (1977), Regeneration of cardiac type mucosa and acquisition of Barrett mucosa after esophagogastrostomy. *Gastroenterology*, **72**, 669–675.

Hamilton, S.R., Hutcheon, D.F., Ravich, W.J. *et al.* (1984), Adenocarcinoma in Barrett's esophagus after elimination of gastroesophageal reflux. *Gastroenterology*, **86**, 356–360.

Hattori, K., Winans, C.S., Archer, F. and Kirsner, J.B. (1974), Endoscopic diagnosis of esophageal inflammation. *Gastrointest. Endosc.*, **20**, 102–104.

Holt, J.M. (1968), Candida infection of the oesophagus. *Gut*, **9**, 227–231.

Huchzermeyer, H., Paul, F., Seifert, E. *et al.* (1976), Endoscopic results in five patients with Crohn's disease of the esophagus. *Endoscopy*, **8**, 75–81.

Ismail-Beigi, F., Horton, P.F. and Pope, C.E. II (1970), Histological consequences of gastroesophageal reflux in man. *Gastroenterology*, **58**, 163–174.

Ismail-Beigi, F. and Pope, C.E. II (1974), Distribution of the histological changes of gastroesophageal reflux in the distal esophagus of man. *Gastroenterology*, **66**, 1109–1113.

Jass, J.R. (1981), Mucin histochemistry of the columnar epithelium of the oesophagus: a retrospective study. *J. Clin. Pathol.*, **34**, 866–870.

Jensen, K.B., Stenderup, A., Thomsen, J.B. and Bichel, J. (1964), Oesophageal moniliasis in malignant neoplastic disease. *Acta Med. Scand.*, **175**, 455–459.

Kaplinsky, N., Neumann, G., Harzahav, Y. and Frankl, O. (1977), Esophageal ulceration in Behçet's syndrome. *Gastrointest. Endosc.*, **23**, 160.

Kaye, M.D. (1977), Postprandial gastro-oesophageal reflux in healthy people. *Gut*, **18**, 709–712.

Kaye, M.D. and Showalter, J.P. (1974), Pyloric incompetence in patients with symptomatic gastroesophageal reflux. *J. Lab. Clin. Med.*, **83**, 198–206.

Kikendall, J.W., Friedman, A.C., Oyewole, M.A. *et al.* (1983), Pill-induced esophageal injury. Case reports and review of the medical literature. *Dig. Dis. Sci.*, **28**, 174–182.

Kobayashi, S. and Kasugai, T. (1974), Endoscopic and biopsy criteria for the diagnosis of esophagitis with a fibreoptic esophagoscope. *Dig. Dis.*, **19**, 345–352.

Kodsi, B.E., Wickremesinghe, P.C., Kozinn, P.J. *et al.* (1976), Candida esophagitis. A prospective study of 27 cases. *Gastroenterology*, **71**, 715–719.

Landres, R.T., Kuster, G.G.R. and Strum, W.B. (1978), Eosinophilic esophagitis in a patient with vigorous achalasia. *Gastroenterology*, **74**, 1298–1301.

Lee, J–H., Neumann, D.A. and Welsh, J.D. (1977), Disseminated histoplasmosis presenting with esophageal symptomatology. *Dig. Dis.*, **22**, 831–834.

Livstone, E.M., Sheahan, D.G.. and Behar, J. (1977), Studies of esophageal epithelial cell proliferation in patients with reflux esophagitis. *Gastroenterology*, **73**, 1315–1319.

Lockhart, J.M., McIntyre, W. and Caperton, E.M. (1976), Esophageal ulceration in Behçet's syndrome. *Ann. Intern. Med.*, **84**, 572–573.

McCallum, R.W., Berkowitz, D.M. and Lerner, E. (1981), Gastric emptying in patients with gastroesophageal reflux. *Gastroenterology*, **80**, 285–291.

McDonald, G.B., Brand, D.L. and Thorning, D.R. (1977), Multiple adenomatous neoplasms arising in columnar-lined (Barrett's) esophagus. *Gastroenterology*, **72**, 1317–1321.

McDonald, G.B., Sullivan, K.M., Schuffler, M.D. *et al.* (1981), Esophageal abnormalities in chronic graft versus host disease in humans. *Gastroenterology*, **80**, 914–921.

McKay, J.S. and Day, D.W. (1983), Herpes simplex oesophagitis. *Histopathology*, **7**, 409–420.

McManus, J.P.A. and Webb, J.N. (1975), A yeast-like infection of the esophagus caused by *Lactobacillus acidophilus*. *Gastroenterology*, **68**, 583–586.

Meyer, W., Vollmar, F. and Bär, W. (1979), Barrett-esophagus following total gastrectomy. A contribution to its pathogenesis. *Endoscopy*, **11**, 121–126.

Mihas, A.A., Slaughter, R.L., Goldman, L.N. and Hirschowitz, B.I. (1976), Double lumen esophagus due to reflux esophagitis with fibrous septum formation. *Gastroenterology*, **71**, 136–137.

Miller, L.J., Thistle, J.L., Payne, W.S. *et al.* (1977), Crohn's disease involving the esophagus and colon. Case report. *Mayo Clin. Proc*, **52**, 35–38.

Mossberg, S.M. (1966), The columnar-lined esophagus (Barrett syndrome): an acquired condition? *Gastroenterology*, **50**, 671–676.

Naef, A.P., Savary, M. and Ozzello, L. (1975), Columnar-lined lower esophagus: an acquired lesion with malignant predisposition. Report on 140 cases of Barrett's esophagus with 12 adenocarcinomas. *J. Thorac. Cardiovasc. Surg.*, **70**, 826–835.

Nash, G. and Ross, J.S. (1974), Herpetic esophagitis: a common cause of esophageal ulceration. *Hum. Pathol.*, **5**, 339–345.

Newburger, P.E., Cassady, J.R. and Jaffe, N. (1978), Esophagitis due to adriamycin and radiation therapy for childhood malignancy. *Cancer*, **42**, 417–423.

Onge, G.St. and Bezahler, G.H. (1982), Giant esophageal ulcer associated with cytomegalovirus. *Gastroenterology*, **83**, 127–130.

Owensby, L.C. and Stammer, J.L. (1978), Esophagitis associated with herpes simplex infection in an immunocompetent host. *Gastroenterology*, **74**, 1305–1306.

Patel, G.K., Clift, S.A., Schaefer, R.A. *et al.* (1982), Resolution of severe dysplastic (Ca *in situ*) changes with regression of columnar epithelium (CE) in Barrett's esophagus (BE) on medical treatment (MT). *Gastroenterology*, **82**, 1147 (abstract).

Paull, A., Trier, J.S., Dalton, M.D. *et al.* (1976), The histologic spectrum of Barrett's esophagus. *N. Engl. J. Med.*, **295**, 476–480.

Polachek, A.A. and Matre, W.J. (1964), Gastrointestinal sarcoidosis. Report of a case involving the esophagus. *Am. J. Dig. Dis.*, **9**, 429–433.

Rabin, M.S., Bremner, C.G., and Botha, J.R. (1980), The reflux gastroesophageal polyp. *Am. J. Gastroenterol*, **73**, 451–453.

Raymond, J.I., Khan, A.H., Cain, L.R. and Ramin, J.E. (1980), Multiple esophagogastric fistulas resulting from reflux esophagitis. *Am. J. Gastroenterol.*, **73**, 430–433.

Savary, M. and Miller, G. (1978), *The Esophagus. Handbook and Atlas of Endoscopy*, Gassmann, Solothurn, p. 160.

Schneider, R.P. and Edwards, W. (1977), Histoplasmosis presenting as an esophageal tumor. *Gastrointest. Endosc.*, **23**, 158–159.

Scott, B.B. and Jenkins, D. (1982), Gastro-oesophageal candidiasis. *Gut*, **23**, 137–139.

Seefeld, U., Krejs, G.J., Siebenmann, R.E. and Blum, A.L. (1977), Esophageal histology in gastroesophageal reflux. Morphometric findings in suction biopsies. *Dig. Dis.*, **22**, 956–964.

Spechler, S.J., Schimmel, E.M., Dalton, J.W. *et al.* (1981), Barrett's epithelium complicating lye ingestion with sparing of the distal esophagus. *Gastroenterology*, **81**, 580–583.

Springer, D.J., DaCosta, L.R. and Beck, I.T. (1979), A syndrome of acute self-limiting ulcerative esophagitis in young adults probably due to herpes simplex virus. *Dig. Dis. Sci.*, **24**, 535–539.

Stadelmann, O., Elster, K. and Kuhn, H.A. (1981), Columnar-lined oesophagus (Barrett's syndrome): congenital or acquired? *Endoscopy*, **13**, 140–147.

Thompson, J.J., Zinsser, K.R. and Enterline, H.T. (1983), Barrett's metaplasia and adenocarcinoma of the esophagus and gastroesophageal junction. *Hum. Pathol*, **14**, 42–61.

Trier, J.S. (1970), Morphology of the epithelium of the distal esophagus in patients with midesophageal peptic strictures. *Gastroenterology*, **58**, 444–461.

Weimann, S., Schargetter, H. and Riedler, L. (1979), Oesophageal tuberculosis. *Zentralbl. Chir.*, **104**, 1072–1076.

Weinstein, W.M., Bogoch, E.R. and Bowes, K.L. (1975), The normal human esophageal mucosa: a histological reappraisal. *Gastroenterology*, **68**, 40–44.

Wesdorp, I.C.E., Bartelsman, J., Schipper, M.E.I. and Tytgat, G.N. (1981), Effect of long-term treatment with cimetidine and antacids in Barrett's oesophagus. *Gut*, **22**, 724–727.

Winter, H.S., Madara, J.L., Stafford, R.J. *et al.* (1982), Intraepithelial eosinophils: a new diagnostic criterion for reflux esophagitis. *Gastroenterology*, **83**, 818–823.

Witt, T.R., Bains, M.S., Zaman, M.B. and Martini, N. (1983), Adenocarcinoma in Barrett's esophagus. *J. Thorac. Cardiovasc. Surg.*, **85**, 337–345.

Wolf, B.S., Marshak, R.H., Som, M.L. and Winkelstein, A. (1955), Peptic esophagitis, peptic ulcer of the esophagus and marginal esophagogastric ulceration. *Gastroenterology*, **29**, 744–766.

4 Cysts, non-neoplastic polyps and tumours of the oesophagus

Benign tumours of the oesophagus are uncommon, may be incidental findings in the course of upper intestinal endoscopy, and are often inaccessible or unsuitable for biopsy. Malignant tumours are by contrast quite common, nearly always symptomatic and constitute a major source of biopsy material from this site. In one reported series of 20 000 endoscopic examinations, 376 oesophageal cancers were diagnosed whereas only seven benign tumours were found (Faivre et al., 1978). Before discussing tumours brief mention will be made of cysts and non-neoplastic polyps of the oesophagus.

4.1 Cysts

Developmental cysts are usually extramural, occurring in the adjacent mediastinum, or are incorporated in the outer wall of the oesophagus, so that they are not a source of biopsy material at endoscopy. Acquired cysts are the result of dilatation of the excretory ducts of the submucosal oesophageal glands and when multiple give rise to a characteristic radiological picture of flask or collar-button shaped outpouchings projecting perpendicularly from the lumen (Mendl et al., 1960; Fromkes et al., 1977), so called intramural pseudodiverticulosis or oesophagitis cystica (Voirol et al., 1973; Piazza and Palma, 1977). The aetiology and pathogenesis of this uncommon condition is not clear. A non-specific oesophagitis has been present in the majority of cases often associated with disorders of oesophageal motility and stricture formation. Dilatation of the latter or treatment of oesophagitis has reversed the process in some cases (Bender and Haddad, 1973; Hammon et al., 1974). Directed biopsies show evidence of oesophagitis and may include dilated excretory ducts. *Candida* organisms have been present in some 8% of cases (Fromkes et al., 1977).

45

4.2   Non-neoplastic polyps

Non-neoplastic polyps are uncommon in the oesophagus. Inflammatory polyps can occur at the lower end as a result of reflux and many of the cases reported as squamous cell papillomas have undoubtedly been of this type (Section 4.3.2(a)). They can also develop in a Barrett's oesophagus at the junction of squamous and columnar epithelia. Fibrous or fibrovascular polyps (Totten *et al.*, 1953; Jang *et al.*, 1969) are interesting lesions of unknown aetiology which can reach an enormous size (Dyke, 1927). The majority are attached by a pedicle to the cricopharyngeal area and cases are reported of regurgitation of these polypoid masses into the mouth. They consist of fibrous tissue, which may be myxomatous, in which there are thin-walled blood vessels. A varying amount of adipose tissue is present and this can be the predominant component (Figs 4.1 and 4.2). Inflammation is usually insignificant except where ulceration of the overlying epithelium has occurred. Even when large they may be missed endoscopically because their surface is similar to normal oesophageal mucosa (Burrell and Toffler, 1973). They have to be differentiated from inflammatory fibroid polyps (inflammatory pseudotumours) which have been described in the oesophagus (LiVolsi and Perzin, 1975), although

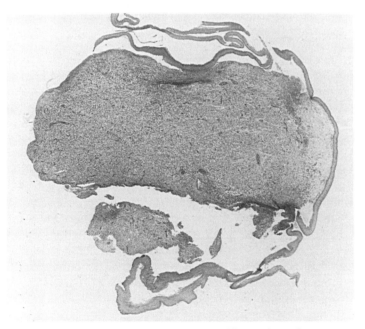

Fig. 4.1   Fibrovascular polyp. Small pedunculated lesion from the upper oesophagus. HE × 14.

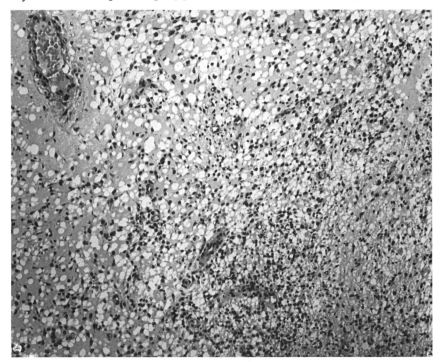

Fig. 4.2 Fibrovascular polyp. The stroma consists of myxomatous and fatty tissue with scattered inflammatory cells and thin-walled blood vessels. HE × 150.

more frequent in the stomach (Section 8.1.5) and elsewhere in the gastro-intestinal tract. These consist of exuberant reparative tissue with a marked inflammatory cell component including eosinophils (Fig. 8.21). They are nearly always associated with sites of ulceration.

The term glycogenic acanthosis has been used to describe plaque-like rather than polypoidal areas which occur particularly in the lower oesophagus. These are discrete, white, round or oval, smooth-surfaced lesions, mostly under 5 mm maximum dimension, which have been observed in up to 15% of upper endoscopies (Bender *et al.*, 1973; Clémençon and Gloor, 1974; Stern *et al.*, 1980). At post-mortem they are almost invariably in the adult oesophagus (Rywlin and Ortega, 1970). Histologically there is hyperplasia of the squamous epithelium with elongation of the papillae and hypertrophy of cells particularly in the superficial layers (Fig. 4.3) which contain abundant glycogen, best demonstrated in alcohol-fixed biopsies. There is no cellular atypia, keratosis or excess parakeratosis and usually no associated inflammation. Although these lesions have no relationship to malignancy their patho-genesis and natural history is not known. Many of the descriptions of

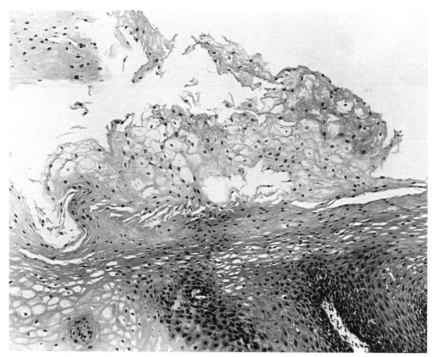

Fig. 4.3   Glycogenic acanthosis. Focal thickening of the squamous epithelium is seen and here the superficial cells are enlarged and pale. HE × 110.

leukoplakia in the oesophagus (Schaer, 1930; Sharp, 1931) were almost certainly describing this condition.

4.3   Benign tumours

From a clinical point of view these may be classified as intramural or intraluminal.

4.3.1   Intramural

Intramural tumours are much the commoner and are predominantly leiomyomas (Totten *et al.*, 1953; Plachta, 1962), although lipomas, neurofibromas, rhabdomyomas (Fig. 4.4), granular cell myoblastomas (Gertsh and Mosimann, 1980) and osteochondromas (Mahour and Harrison, 1967) can also occur. Endoscopically they present as curved or rounded indentations of the oesophageal wall with a freely mobile overlying intact mucosa. Biopsy is contra-indicated except where irregularity or ulceration suggests malignancy (Fig. 4.5). The reasons for this are that

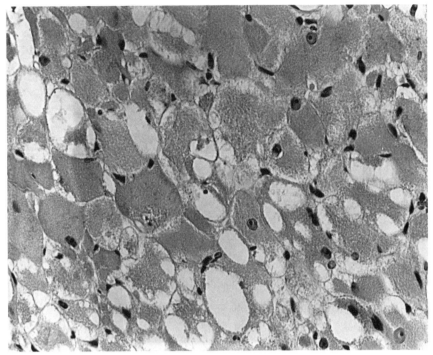

Fig. 4.4 Rhabdomyoma. Sheets of large cells with granular cytoplasm. This very rare tumour was present in the upper oesophagus. HE × 375.

diagnostic material is rarely obtained, the biopsy consisting of mucosa only, and that subsequent surgical enucleation, if indicated, is more difficult as a result of fibrous adhesion of the tumour to the mucosa following healing at the biopsy site. Epithelial hyperplasia of the mucosa overlying a granular cell myoblastoma can result in a superficial resemblance to a well-differentiated squamous cell carcinoma (Gloor and Clémençon, 1975).

4.3.2 Intraluminal

Intraluminal tumours may be either pedunculated or sessile. Occasionally leiomyomas or other benign mesenchymal tumours arising in the submucosa can present as pedunculated lesions and be removed endoscopically. Benign epithelial tumours are extremely uncommon and comprise squamous cell papillomas and adenomas.

(a) *Squamous cell papilloma*. These rare tumours are multilobulated with a granular or warty surface and a firm consistency. They can arise

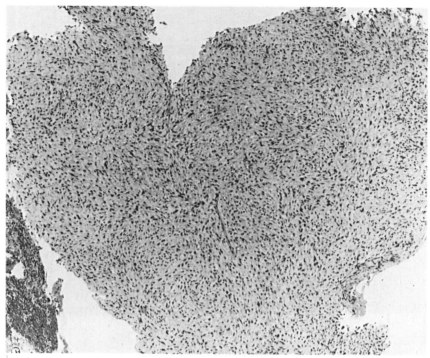

Fig. 4.5 Smooth muscle tumour. Sheets of interlacing spindle cells with only minor pleomorphism. Material was taken from a large ulcerated tumour of the mid-oesophagus which was clinically malignant. Examination of the resection specimen confirmed this. HE × 60.

anywhere in the oesophagus although the majority of cases have been in the lower third. Most have been under 1.5 cm in diameter and have occurred in men (Zeabart *et al.*, 1979). Sometimes multiple lesions have been present (Parnell *et al.*, 1978). Histologically they have a papillary architecture with central cores of vascular connective tissue covered by acanthotic stratified squamous epithelium which lacks atypia and shows normal differentiation from the basal to the surface layers (Fig. 4.6). They have to be differentiated from inflammatory polyps occurring in association with gastro-oesophageal reflux (Staples *et al.*, 1978; Rabin *et al.*, 1980). These show basal cell hyperplasia with varying erosion of the epithelium and often a marked acute inflammatory cell infiltrate in the lamina propria and have a relatively smooth surface (Fig. 4.7). There is no evidence that squamous cell papillomas are pre-malignant.

(b) *Adenoma.* The only situation where bona fide examples of adenomatous lesions have been described has been in the columnar-lined

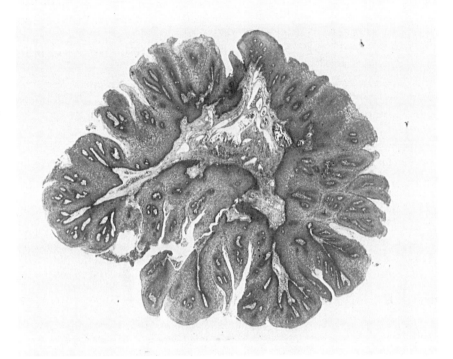

Fig. 4.6 Squamous cell papilloma. Projections of hyperplastic squamous cells with connective tissue core. HE × 16.

(Barrett's) oesophagus (McDonald *et al.*, 1977) where dysplasia in this pre-malignant condition may result in polypoid masses with a tubular or villous configuration (Section 3.2.2). Intervening non-polypoid mucosa may also show dysplasia.

A villous adenoma which had undergone malignant change has been reported in a colon bypass after oesophageal resection for cancer (Goldsmith and Beattie, 1968).

4.4   Malignant tumours

Carcinoma of the oesophagus is a disease with a very marked variation in incidence even within relatively small geographical areas, such as along the southern shore of the Caspian Sea (Mahboubi *et al.*, 1973) and in northern China (Co-ordinating Group, 1973). Its high mortality is related to the fact that by the time symptoms develop the tumour is usually large and local invasion of the oesophagus and surrounding tissues is advanced. There is often a history of heavy smoking and/or alcohol consumption. In approximately 5% of cases an associated condition such as achalasia (Pierce *et al.*, 1970), the Plummer-Vinson syndrome (Wynder *et al.*, 1957), a long-standing stricture following ingestion of corrosives (Appelqvist and Salmo, 1980), a columnar-lined oesophagus secondary to reflux oesophagitis (Section 3.2), or a diverticulum is present. Occasionally families have been described with late-onset keratosis palmaris et plantaris (tylosis), inherited as an autosomal dominant, in which there has been a very high prevalence of cancer of the oesophagus (Howel-Evans *et al.*, 1958; Shine and Allison, 1966).

Malignant non-epithelial tumours rarely occur in the oesophagus and occasionally tumours spread directly or metastasize to the oesophagus from other sites and give rise to symptoms.

4.4.1 *Squamous cell carcinoma*

This accounts for over 90% of primary malignant tumours of the oesophagus (Table 4.1). Macroscopically they appear as exophytic, ulcerating or infiltrating lesions or a combination of these, and often result in a stricture

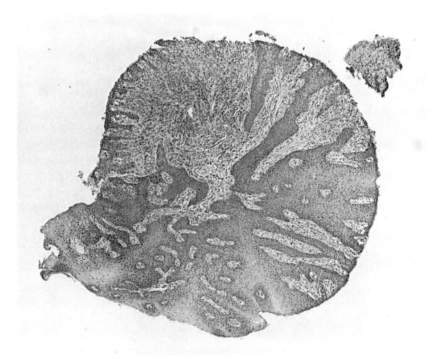

Fig. 4.7 Inflammatory polyp. One of several smooth surfaced polyps at the lower end of the oesophagus in a patient with reflux oesophagitis. HE × 40.

Table 4.1 Different types of primary malignant tumours of the oesophagus where histology was available seen at the Memorial Hospital, New York, between the years 1926–1968 (Turnbull *et al.*, 1973)

Type	Number	Percentage
Squamous cell carcinoma (SCC)	1618	93.0
SCC with glandular features	5	0.3
SCC with spindle cell metaplasia	5	0.3
Adenocarcinoma	45	2.6
Mucoepidermoid carcinoma	1	0.05
Leiomyosarcoma	7	0.4
Oat cell tumour	1	0.05
Malignant melanoma	2	0.1
Unclassified	55	3.2
Total	1739	100

which is usually irregular, friable and haemorrhagic. However, undermining of proximal adjacent epithelium by the tumour may give rise to a smooth annular stenosis. A stricture may be passed only with smaller instruments, and brush cytology in addition to multiple biopsies should always be carried out in these circumstances. In some instances it is necessary to dilate a stricture before satisfactory samples can be obtained, or for biopsies to be taken blindly by passing only the forceps through the strictured site.

A considerable range of microscopical appearances may be seen even in biopsies from the same tumour. In the best differentiated tumours keratinization occurs in individual cells or towards the centre of nests of atypical squamous cells and intercellular bridges may be evident (Fig. 4.8). With less differentiated tumours the amount of cytoplasm decreases and the cells become spheroidal. Sometimes a superficial resemblance to a basal cell carcinoma may be present when cells adjoining the stroma have a palisaded arrangement (Fig. 4.9). Apart from the degree of differentiation the amount of stroma is quite variable as well as its inflammatory cell content. Occasionally the only evidence of malignancy in a biopsy is the presence of tumour cells in the lymphatics (Fig. 4.10). In most cases the diagnosis of squamous cell carcinoma is reasonably straightforward. However, regenerating epithelium in a biopsy from the edge of a benign ulcer or erosion (Fig. 4.11) may show considerable enlargement of the basal and parabasal cells with numerous mitoses and, particularly in poorly orientated material, give a misleading impression of malignancy. Lack of pleomorphism, uniformity of nuclear morphology and the tendency towards normal surface maturation are all helpful pointers to a reactive rather than a neoplastic state. The presence and

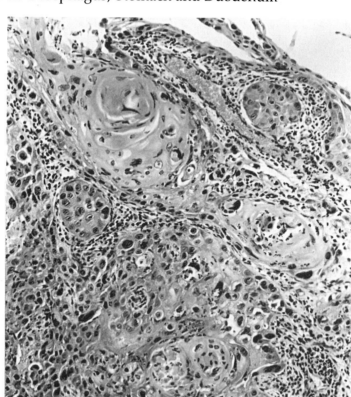

Fig. 4.8   Well-differentiated squamous cell carcinoma with central keratinization in many of the cell clumps. HE × 150.

degree of active inflammation is of some value although this can be a prominent feature in some cancers.

Two variants of squamous cell carcinoma, verrucous squamous cell carcinoma and so-called carcinosarcoma, deserve special mention in that although both are rare, they may give rise to misleading appearances in biopsy material.

(a) *Verrucous squamous cell carcinoma.* This is usually a large, exophytic, slowly growing neoplasm which rarely metastasizes and which has a shaggy papillary or warty shape. Similar tumours occur at other sites notably the oral cavity, larynx, glans penis, vulva and anal canal (Kraus and Perez-Mesa, 1966; Prioleau *et al.*, 1980). Most of the cases in the

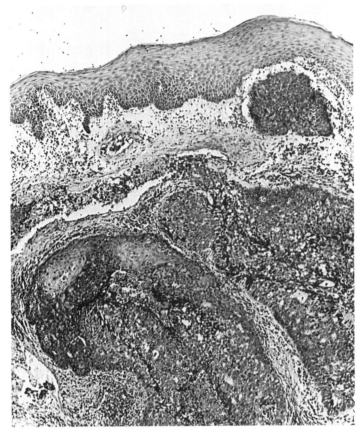

Fig. 4.9 Poorly differentiated squamous cell carcinoma underlying intact oesophageal epithelium. 'Basal cell' features are apparent in some areas. HE × 60.

oesophagus have occurred in the upper part (Minielly *et al.*, 1967). In some there has been a history of achalasia, diverticulum (Minielly *et al.*, 1967) or lye stricture (Parkinson *et al.*, 1970). Histologically there are papillary projections composed of well-differentiated squamous cells with parakeratosis and hyperkeratosis most prominent between the papillae (Figs 4.12 and 4.13). In biopsies, evidence of invasion is often lacking so that a pathologist unaware of the endoscopic appearance would interpret the rather bland appearances as a benign hyperplastic process.

(b) *Carcinosarcoma.* These usually occur as bulky polypoid growths in the lower oesophagus. Histologically they consist of a 'sarcomatous' component of interlacing bundles of spindle-shaped cells in which bizarre

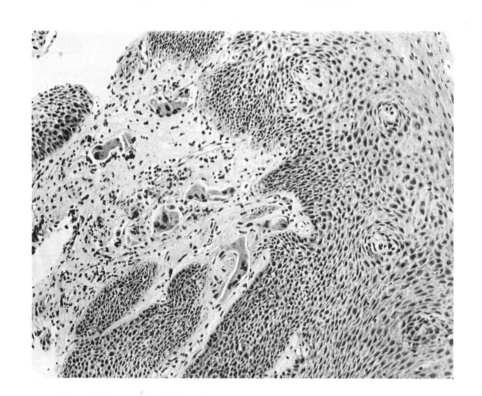

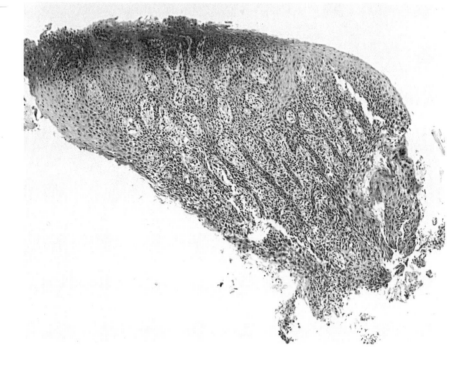

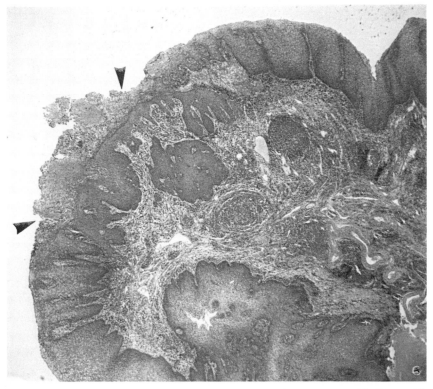

Fig. 4.12 Verrucous carcinoma. Markedly thickened squamous epithelium with minimal atypia and focal surface keratinization (arrowed). The biopsy came from the edge of a large exophytic clinically malignant tumour of the mid-oesophagus. HE × 22.

giant cells are present, and in which osteoid and cartilaginous metaplasia may occur, together with an epithelial component of squamous or undifferentiated carcinoma (Fig. 4.14). Occasionally an adeno-carcinomatous (du Boulay and Isaacson, 1981) or adenocystic component (Talbert and Cantrell, 1963) has also been described. There may be an admixture of these two elements throughout the tumour or the sarcomatous part may predominate with often only inconspicuous intramucosal or invasive squamous cell carcinoma confined to small areas

Fig. 4.10 Poorly differentiated squamous carcinoma cells in subepithelial lymphatics. Biopsy from a mid-oesophageal stricture. HE × 150.

Fig. 4.11 In this tangentially sectioned biopsy there is a resemblance to an infiltrating carcinoma, but surface maturation and a heavy inflammatory infiltrate are in keeping with the epithelial changes being reactive and not neoplastic. HE × 60.

at the base of the pedicle. With this latter appearance the term pseudosarcoma has been used in the belief that the spindle cell element represents a non-neoplastic reparative host response to the carcinoma. The finding of transition from typical squamous carcinoma to the sarcomatous component when carefully looked for in many of the resected specimens (Smith and Gowing, 1953; Talbert and Cantrell, 1963) and the demonstration ultrastructurally of tonofibrils and well-developed desmosomes in some of the spindle cells (Osamura *et al.*, 1978; du Boulay and Isaacson, 1981) together with evidence of collagen production (Battifora, 1976) suggests that the 'sarcomatous' cells are squamous cells which have undergone mesenchymal metaplasia. Biopsy of these tumours may

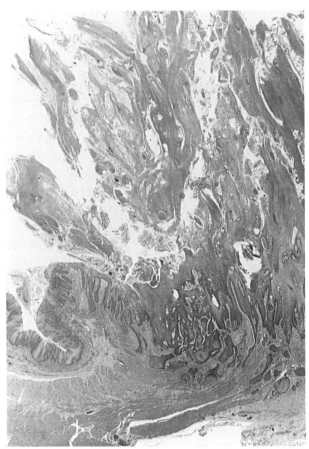

Fig. 4.13   Verrucous carcinoma. A section from the resected specimen shows the papillary surface of the tumour and obvious invasion of the oesophageal wall. HE × 6.

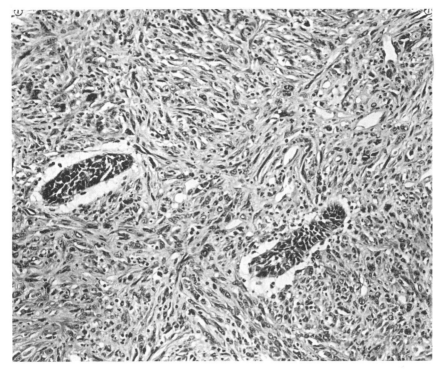

Fig. 4.14   Carcinosarcoma. Two groups of poorly differentiated squamous cell carcinoma surrounded by 'sarcomatous' tissue composed of spindle cells with marked nuclear irregularity, hyperchromasia and mitotic activity. In other areas gradations between these two patterns were apparent. HE × 150.

produce tissue suggesting a highly malignant undifferentiated sarcoma although in the majority of reported cases and in two personally studied examples squamous cell carcinoma of varying degrees of differentiation has been present. In some of the reports this tumour has been associated with longer survival than the usual type of squamous cell carcinoma (Talbert and Cantrell, 1963), whereas in others the prognosis has appeared similar (du Boulay and Isaacson, 1981).

4.4.2 Superficial (early) oesophageal carcinoma

There are increasing reports of oesophageal cancer in which the tumour is confined to the mucosa or has spread no further than the submucosa. Most emanate from China or Japan (Ide *et al.*, 1976; Chinese authors, 1977) although cases are also beginning to appear in the European literature (Seifert *et al.*, 1973; Miller *et al.*, 1979; Barge *et al.*, 1981). In China the majority of cases have been picked up in mass surveys involving cytology and X-ray examinations in high incidence areas, but other cases have been symptomatic. At endoscopy, lesions have been plaque-like or showed single or multiple map-like erosions which can resemble the changes in reflux oesophagitis but, unlike that condition, are usually separated by normal appearing mucosa from the gastro-oesophageal junction. Less commonly a protuberant lesion is present. Occasionally the mucosa has appeared normal apart from a colour change (occult type) and histological examination of resected specimens has shown these to be intraepithelial carcinomas. Apart from the latter, biopsies from these lesions usually show invasive squamous cell carcinoma.

Like carcinoma of the cervix, most cases of oesophageal carcinoma almost certainly arise on the basis of preceding dysplasia of the squamous epithelium. Varying degrees of this are quite commonly present in resection specimens of advanced oesophageal carcinoma when the mucosa around the tumour is extensively sampled (Fig. 4.15), and

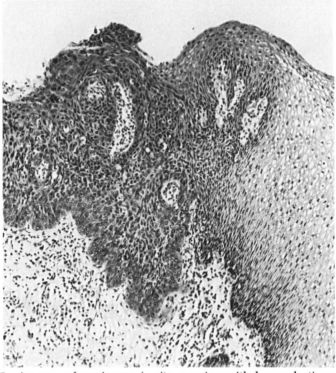

Fig. 4.15 An area of carcinoma *in situ* merging with hyperplastic squamous epithelium (right). HE × 114.

screening of high-risk populations (Figs. 4.16 and 4.17) and high-risk groups such as those with tylosis (Fig. 4.18) will detect these changes in oesophageal biopsy samples.

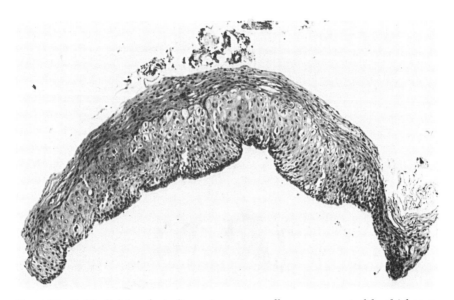

Fig. 4.16 Epithelial dysplasia. Large immature cells occupy most of the thickness of the epithelium. Biopsy taken as part of a field study in northern China. HE × 72.

4.4.3 Adenocarcinoma

As the cardio-oesophageal junction is approached an increasing proportion of biopsies of malignant tissue will consist of adenocarcinoma. The majority of these are tumours that have originated in the stomach, particularly from the cardiac region, and spread upwards, often undermining the squamous epithelium of the oesophagus (Fig. 4.19). A variety of histological appearances are seen including signet-ring cells and well-differentiated glandular tumours. The latter have to be differentiated from superficial oesophageal (cardiac) glands, which are often present in biopsies from this region. There can be an intimate admixture of glandular tissue with the basal layer of the squamous epithelium in neoplastic and inflammatory conditions at this site and distinction between the two may be very difficult (Figs 4.20, 4.21 and 4.22). In such circumstances repeat endoscopy with multiple biopsies may be necessary.

Primary adenocarcinomas of the oesophagus are much less common. It is probable that nearly all of them arise in a columnar-lined (Barrett's) oesophagus (Section 3.2) and biopsy material from the oesophagus may include adjacent Barrett's type mucosa (Figs 4.23 and 4.24). Carcinomas with adenoid cystic differentiation are rare (Epstein *et al.*, 1984). Most have occurred in the middle part of the oesophagus with approximately

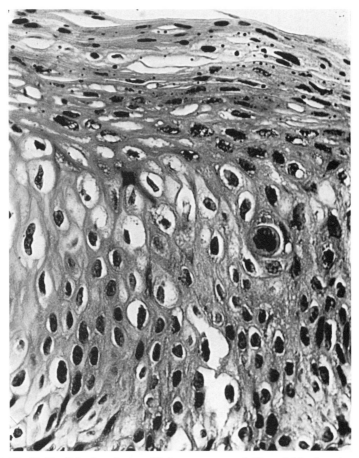

Fig. 4.17 Epithelial dysplasia. Higher power of Fig. 4.16 showing large dyskaryotic cell high in the epithelium. Surface differentiation is apparent with layers of parakeratotic cells some of which contain keratohyalin granules. HE × 375.

Fig. 4.18 Questionable epithelial dysplasia is present in this mid-oesophageal biopsy from a patient with tylosis and a family history of oesophageal carcinoma. There is focal attenuation of the epithelium and deeply staining epithelial cells are present in some areas in the absence of any associated inflammation. HE × 150.

Fig. 4.19 Moderately well-differentiated adenocarcinoma present beneath oesophageal epithelium and in places breaching it. HE × 41.

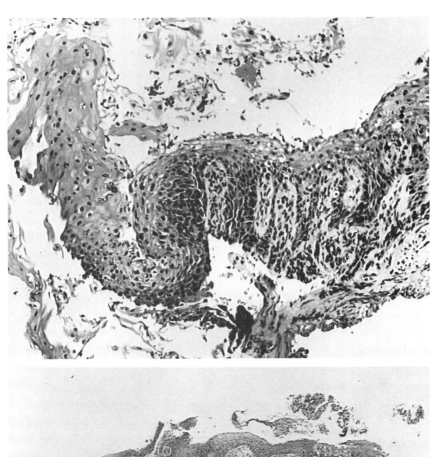

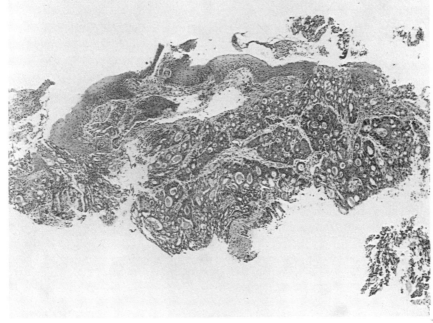

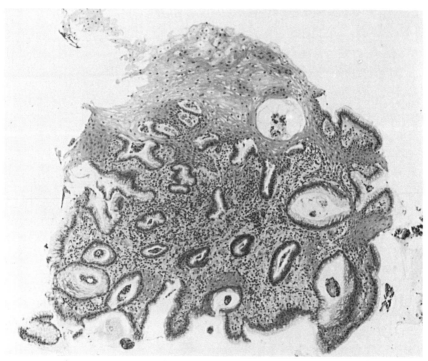

Fig. 4.20 Biopsy from the cardio-oesophageal junction showing intimate admixture of squamous and glandular epithelium. There is a moderate inflammatory infiltrate in the lamina propria. HE × 60.

equal numbers of males and females affected. Characteristically the tumour bulges into the oesophagus and is covered by more or less intact epithelium. Histologically, rounded masses of uniform small epithelial cells are seen arranged in anastomosing cords and as solid sheets in which pseudocysts may occur (Fig. 4.25). Hyaline material which is PAS positive and alcianophilic is present between the trabeculae and in the cystic spaces, and consists of replicated basement membrane on ultrastructural examination. The histogenesis of this tumour is debated but an origin from the intercalated ducts of the submucosal glands appears likely

Fig. 4.21 A higher power of Fig. 4.20 shows normal mucin-secreting glandular epithelium without atypia closely applied to the deep surface of squamous epithelium. HE × 150.

Fig. 4.22 Obviously neoplastic glands of a moderately well-differentiated adenocarcinoma underlie oesophageal epithelium in this biopsy from a stricture at the lower end of the oesophagus. Direct spread from a gastric primary. HE × 120.

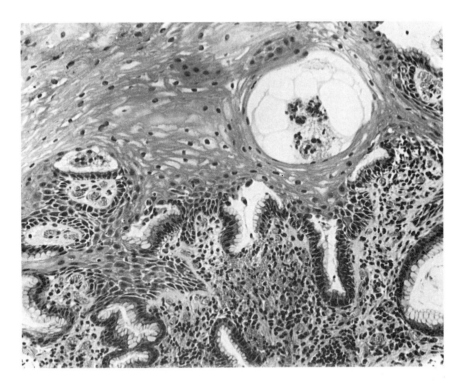

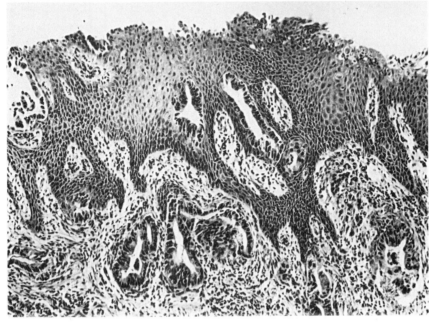

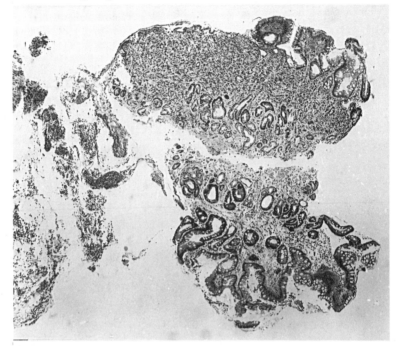

Fig. 4.23   Adenocarcinoma in columnar-lined oesophagus. The upper piece of tissue is infiltrated by malignant cells. HE × 38.

(Sweeney and Cooney, 1980). Its behaviour is more aggressive than its salivary gland and bronchial counterparts and the average length of survival after operation has been seven months.

A few examples of mucoepidermoid carcinoma of the oesophagus have also been described (Azzopardi and Menzies, 1962; Kay, 1968; Weitzner, 1970).

4.4.4   Oat cell carcinoma

Since the first description of primary oat cell carcinoma of the oesophagus (McKeown, 1952) approximately 50 cases have been reported. A recent review of a large series of primary oesophageal carcinomas identified 2.4% of the total with this morphology (Briggs and Ibrahim, 1983). The tumours presumably arise from argyrophil cells which have been identified in the basal layer of the oesophageal epithelium (Tateishi *et al.*, 1974), and in some tumours a high adrenocorticotrophic hormone (ACTH) content has been recorded (Tateishi *et al.*, 1976). Unlike similar tumours in the lung many have occurred in females (Briggs and Ibrahim, 1983). In the majority of cases these tumours have been large, often protuberant and occurred in the middle and lower thirds of the oesophagus. Histologically, small fusiform or polygonal cells with little cytoplasm and hyperchromatic nuclei are present which are arranged in sheets or as anastomosing cords and ribbons (Fig. 4.26). Crush artefact of the tumour cells is common particularly in biopsy material. Rosette formation may be present and in some cases tubular or acinar differentiation is seen. A few tumours have shown a squamous component (McKeown, 1952; Rosen *et al.*, 1975; Cook *et al.*, 1976). If spread from the lung can be ruled out (Delpre *et al.*, 1980), confirmation that the tumour is a primary oat cell carcinoma and not an undifferentiated squamous cell carcinoma or

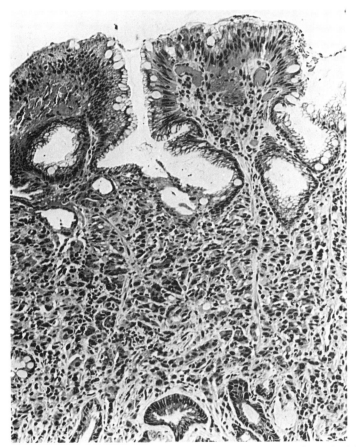

Fig. 4.24   Detail of Fig. 4.23 with individual and small clumps of poorly differentiated adenocarcinoma cells infiltrating the lamina propria. Note goblet cells in surface and glandular epithelium which shows an incomplete type of intestinal metaplasia often seen in this type of mucosa. HE × 159.

lymphoma depends on the demonstration of argyrophilia of the tumour cells or, more definitively, the finding of neurosecretory granules on ultrastructural examination. Although the prognosis is poor it is important to diagnose this tumour since, as with small cell carcinoma of the bronchus, multi-agent chemotherapy and radiation rather than surgery is the treatment of choice (Kelsen *et al.*, 1980; Rosenthal and Lemkin, 1983).

4.4.5 Malignant melanoma

Primary malignant melanomas of the oesophagus are very uncommon with approximately 30 well-documented cases in the world literature. They presumably are derived from melanoblasts in the epithelium of the

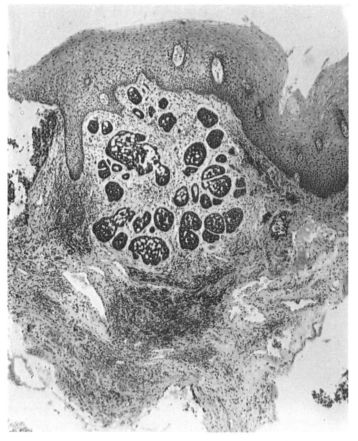

Fig. 4.25 Adenocystic carcinoma. Groups of cells with a cribriform pattern beneath intact oesophageal epithelium. HE × 60.

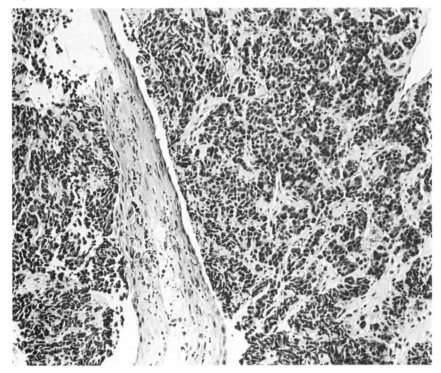

Fig. 4.26 Oat cell carcinoma. Groups and strands of small cells with scanty cytoplasm and intersected by fibrous tissue. Some crush artefact is seen focally. HE × 150.

oesophagus, which have been found in 4% of oesophagi examined at post-mortem (De la Pava *et al.*, 1963). Characteristically the tumours are large, polypoid, friable and may or may not be pigmented. The commonest site is the middle third of the oesophagus. In a few cases the adjacent mucosa has shown patchy or diffuse melanosis (Sakornpant *et al.*, 1964; Piccone *et al.*, 1970). Satellite lesions may be present (Musher and Lindner, 1974). To be acceptable as a primary melanoma the tumour should be seen to arise from, or be surrounded by, squamous epithelium showing junctional change (Raven and Dawson, 1964) and this may only be apparent in resected material (Fig. 4.27). The prognosis of this tumour is poor.

Involvement of the oesophagus by metastasis from a malignant melanoma usually results in compression of the lumen so that at endoscopy a smooth projecting lesion covered by intact mucosa is seen and biopsies may not sample the tumour (Butler *et al.*, 1975).

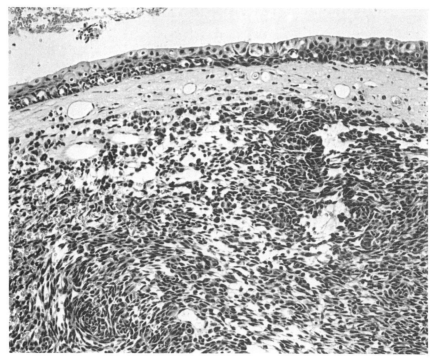

Fig. 4.27 Malignant melanoma. Spindle cells deep to flattened oesophageal epithelium in which there is junctional change. HE × 150.

4.4.6 *Secondary tumours*

Apart from the direct spread of a tumour from gastric and bronchial primaries, secondary deposits in the oesophagus may result from lymphatic or blood stream spread. Metastatic breast carcinoma in the submucosal lymphatics of the oesophagus or adjacent mediastinal lymph nodes usually results in concentric stenosis of the mid-oesophagus with an intact mucosa seen endoscopically. Because of this, biopsies may be non-contributory (Polk *et al.*, 1967). Blood stream spread from primary tumours in the testis, prostate (Gross and Freedman, 1942), kidney (Nussbaum and Grossman, 1976) and pancreas have occasionally been reported.

Oesophageal involvement occurs rarely in Hodgkin's disease either by compression or due to infiltration from affected mediastinal lymph nodes (Bichel, 1951) and dysphagia can be the presenting symptom (Strauch *et al.*, 1971; Stein *et al.*, 1981). This may also occur with non-Hodgkin's lymphomas (Givler, 1970) and there is a case report of a primary histiocytic lymphoma of this site (Berman *et al.*, 1979). Apparent primary extramedullary plasmacytomas of the oesophagus have also been described (Morris and Pead, 1972; Ahmed *et al.*, 1976).

References

Ahmed, N., Ramos, S., Sika, J. *et al.* (1976), Primary extramedullary esophageal plasmacytoma. First case report. *Cancer*, **38**, 943–947.

Appelqvist, P. and Salmo, M. (1980), Lye corrosion carcinoma of the esophagus. A review of 63 cases. *Cancer*, **45**, 2655–2658.

Azzopardi, J.G. and Menzies, T. (1962), Primary oesophageal adenocarcinoma. Confirmation of its existence by the finding of mucous gland tumours. *Br. J. Surg.*, **49**, 497–506.

Barge, J., Molas, G., Maillard, J.N. *et al.* (1981), Superficial oesophageal carcinoma: an oesophageal counterpart of early gastric cancer. *Histopathology*, **5**, 499–510.

Battifora, H. (1976), Spindle cell carcinoma. Ultrastructural evidence of squamous origin and collagen production by the tumour cells. *Cancer*, **37**, 2275–2282.

Bender, M.D., Allison, J., Cuartas, F. and Montgomery, C. (1973), Glycogenic acanthosis of the esophagus: a form of benign epithelial hyperplasia. *Gastroenterology*, **65**, 373–380.

Bender, M.D. and Haddad, J.K. (1973), Disappearance of multiple esophageal diverticula following treatment of esophagitis: serial endoscopic, manometric, and radiologic observations. *Gastrointest. Endosc.*, **20**, 19–22.

Berman, M.D., Falchuk, K.R., Trey, C. and Gramm, H.F. (1979), Primary histiocytic lymphoma of the esophagus. *Dig. Dis. Sci.*, **24**, 883–886.

Bichel, J. (1951), Hodgkin's disease of the oesophagus. *Acta Radiol. (Stockh.)*, **35**, 371–374.

Briggs, J.C. and Ibrahim, N.B.N. (1983), Oat cell carcinoma of the oesophagus: a clinico-pathological study of 23 cases. *Histopathology*, **7**, 261–277.

Burrell, M. and Toffler, R. (1973), Fibrovascular polyp of the esophagus. *Dig. Dis.*, **18**, 714–718.

Butler, M.L., Vantheertum, R.L. and Teplick, S.K. (1975), Metastatic malignant melanoma of the esophagus: a case report. *Gastroenterology*, **69**, 1334–1337.

Chinese authors. (1977), Pathology of early esophageal squamous cell carcinoma. *Chinese Med. J.*, **3**, 180–193.

Clémençon, G. and Gloor, F. (1974), Benign epithelial hyperplasia of the esophagus: glycogenic acanthosis. *Endoscopy*, **6**, 214–217.

Cook, M.G., Eusebi, V. and Betts, C.M. (1976), Oat-cell carcinoma of the oesophagus: a recently recognized entity. *J. Clin. Pathol.*, **29**, 1068–1073.

Co-ordinating Group for Research of Esophageal Carcinoma, Chinese Academy of Medical Sciences and Honan Province (1973), The early detection of carcinoma of the esophagus. *Sci. Sin.*, **16**, 457–463.

De la Pava, S., Nigogosyan, G., Pickren, J.W. and Cabreras, A. (1963), Melanosis of the esophagus. *Cancer*, **16**, 48–50.

Delpre, G., Kadish, U., Glanz, I. and Avidor, I. (1980), Endoscopic biopsy diagnosis of oat cell carcinoma of the lung penetrating the esophagus. *Gastrointest. Endosc.*, **26**, 104–106.

du Boulay, C.E.H. and Isaacson, P. (1981), Carcinoma of the oesophagus with spindle cell features. *Histopathology*, **5**, 403–414.

Dyke, S.C. (1927), Benign polyp of the oesophagus of great size. *J. Pathol.*, **30**, 309–312.

Epstein, J.I., Sears, D.L., Tucker, R.S. and Eagan, J.W.Jr. (1984), Carcinoma of the esophagus with adenoid cystic differentiation. *Cancer*, **53**, 1131–1136.

Faivre, J., Bory, R. and Moulinier, B. (1978), Benign tumors of oesophagus: value of endoscopy. *Endoscopy*, **10**, 264–268.

Fromkes, J., Thomas, F.B., Mekhjian, H. *et al.* (1977), Esophageal intramural pseudodiverticulosis. *Dig. Dis.*, **22**, 690–700.

Gertsch, Ph. and Mosimann, R. (1980), A rare tumour of the esophagus: the granular cell myoblastoma. Report of a case and review of the literature. *Endoscopy*, **12**, 245–249.

Givler, R.L. (1970), Esophageal lesions in leukaemia and lymphoma. *Am. J. Dig. Dis.*, **15**, 31–36.

Gloor, F. and Clémençon, G. (1975), Granular cell tumors ('myoblastomas') of the esophagus. *Endoscopy*, **7**, 239–242.

Goldsmith, H.S. and Beattie, E.J.Jr. (1968), Malignant villous tumour in a colon bypass. *Ann. Surg.*, **167**, 98–100.

Gross, P. and Freedman, L.J. (1942), Obstructing secondary carcinoma of the esophagus. *Arch. Pathol.*, **33**, 361–364.

Hammon, J.W.Jr., Rice, R.P., Postlethwait, R.W. and Young, W.G. (1974), Esophageal intramural diverticulosis: a clinical and pathological survey. *Ann. Thorac. Surg.*, **17**, 260–267.

Howel-Evans, W., McConnell, R.B., Clarke, C.A. and Sheppard, P.M. (1958), Carcinoma of the oesophagus with keratosis palmaris et plantaris (tylosis). A study of two families. *Q. J. Med.*, **27**, 413–429.

Ide H., Endo, M., Kinoshita, Y. *et al.* (1976), Clinicopathological aspect of superficial esophageal cancer (22 cases of our experience). *Chir. Gastroenterol.*, **10**, 9–15.

Jang, G.C., Clouse, M.E. and Fleischner, F.G. (1969), Fibrovascular polyp: a benign intraluminal tumor of the esophagus. *Radiology*, **92**, 1196–1200.

Kay, S. (1968), Mucoepidermoid carcinoma of the esophagus. Report of two cases. *Cancer*, **22**, 1053–1059.

Kelsen, D.P., Weston, E., Kurtz, R. *et al.* (1980), Small-cell carcinoma of the esophagus. Treatment by chemotherapy alone. *Cancer*, **45**, 1558–1561.

Kraus, T.K. and Perez-Mesa, C. (1966), Verrucous carcinoma: clinical and pathologic study of 105 cases involving oral cavity, larynx and genitalia. *Cancer*, **19**, 26–38.

LiVolsi, V.A. and Perzin, K.H. (1975), Inflammatory pseudotumors (inflammatory fibrous polyps) of the esophagus. A clinicopathologic study. *Dig. Dis.*, **20**, 475–481.

McDonald, G.B., Brand, D.L. and Thorning, D.R. (1977), Multiple adenomatous neoplasms arising in columnar-lined (Barrett's) esophagus. *Gastroenterology*, **72**, 1317–1321.

McKeown F. (1952), Oat-cell carcinoma of the oesophagus. *J. Pathol. Bacteriol.*, **64**, 889–891.

Mahboubi, E., Kmet, J., Cook, P.J. *et al.* (1973), Oesophageal cancer studies in the Caspian littoral of Iran: the Caspian cancer registry. *Br. J. Cancer*, **28**, 197–214.

Mahour, G.H. and Harrison, E.G.Jr. (1967), Osteochondroma (tracheobronchial choristoma) of the esophagus. Report of a case. *Cancer*, **20**, 1489–1493.

Mendl, K., McKay, J.M. and Tanner, C.H. (1960), Intramural diverticulosis of the oesophagus and Rokitansky-Aschoff sinuses in the gall-bladder. *Br. J. Radiol.*, **33**, 496–501.

Miller, G., Maurer, W., Savary, M. *et al.* (1979), A case of oesophageal cancer limited to the mucosa and submucosa. *Endoscopy*, **3**, 175–178.

Minielly, J.A., Harrison, E.G.Jr., Fontana, R.S. and Payne, W.S. (1967), Verrucous squamous cell carcinoma of the esophagus. *Cancer*, **20**, 2078–2087.

Morris, W.T. and Pead, J.L. (1972), Myeloma of the oesophagus. *J. Clin. Pathol.*, **25**, 537–538.

Musher, D.R. and Lindner, A.E. (1974), Primary melanoma of the esophagus. *Dig. Dis.*, **19**, 855–859.

Nussbaum, M. and Grossman, M. (1976), Metastases to the esophagus causing gastrointestinal bleeding. *Am. J. Gastroenterol.*, **66**, 467–472.

Osamura, R.Y., Watanabe, K., Shimamura, K. *et al.* (1978), Polypoid carcinoma of the esophagus. A unifying term for 'carcinosarcoma' and 'pseudosarcoma'. *Am. J. Surg. Pathol.*, **2**, 201–208.

Parkinson, A.T., Haidak, G.L. and McInerney, R.P. (1970), Verrucous squamous cell carcinoma of the esophagus following lye stricture. *Chest*, **57**, 489–492.

Parnell, S.A.C., Peppercorn, M.A., Antonioli, D.A. *et al.* (1978), Squamous cell papilloma of the esophagus. Report of a case after peptic esophagitis and repeated bougienage with review of the literature. *Gastroenterology*, **74**, 910–913.

Piazza, M. and Palma, P.D. (1977), Polycystic 'dystrophy' of the esophagus. *Am. J. Clin. Pathol.*, **67**, 307. (Letter).

Piccone, V.A., Klopstock, R., LeVeen, H.H. and Sika, J. (1970), Primary malignant melanoma of the esophagus associated with melanosis of the entire esophagus. First case report. *J. Thorac. Cardiovasc. Surg.*, **59**, 864–870.

Pierce, W.S., MacVaugh, H. III. and Johnson, J. (1970), Carcinoma of the esophagus arising in patients with achalasia of the cardia. *J. Thorac. Cardiovasc. Surg.*, **59**, 335–339.

Plachta, A. (1962), Benign tumors of the esophagus. Review of literature and report of 99 cases. *Am. J. Gastroenterol.*, **38**, 639–652.

Polk, H.C.Jr., Camp, F.A. and Walker, A.W. (1967), Dysphagia and esophageal stenosis. Manifestation of metastatic mammary cancer. *Cancer*, **20**, 2002–2007.

Prioleau, P.G., Santa Cruz, D.J., Meyer, J.S. and Bauer, W.C. (1980), Verrucous carcinoma. A light and electron microscopic, autoradiographic, and immunofluorescence study. *Cancer*, **45**, 2849–2857.

Rabin, M.S., Bremner, C.G. and Botha, J.R. (1980), The reflux gastroesophageal polyp. *Am. J. Gastroenterol.*, **73**, 451–453.

Raven, R.W. and Dawson, I. (1964), Malignant melanoma of the oesophagus. *Br. J. Surg.*, **51**, 551–555.

Rosen, Y., Moon, S. and Kim, B. (1975), Small cell epidermoid carcinoma of the esophagus. An oat-cell-like carcinoma. *Cancer*, **36**, 1042–1049.

Rosenthal, S.N. and Lemkin, J.A. (1983), Multiple small cell carcinomas of the esophagus. *Cancer*, **51**, 1944–1946.

Rywlin, A.M. and Ortega, R. (1970), Glycogenic acanthosis of the esophagus. *Arch. Pathol.*, **90**, 439–443.

Sakornpant, P., Barlow, D. and Bevan, C.M. (1964). Two cases of primary malignant melanoma of the oesophagus. *Br. J. Surg.*, **51**, 386–388.

Schaer, H. (1930), Systematische untersuchungen über das vorkommen von vorstadien des krebses in der menschlichen speiseröhre. *Z. Krebsforsch.*, **31**, 217–253.

Seifert, E., Borst, H.H., Ostertag, H. *et al.* (1973), Carcinoma *in situ* of the esophagus (early esophageal cancer). A case report and a review of the literature. *Endoscopy*, **5**, 147–153.

Sharp, G.S. (1931), Leokoplakia of the esophagus. *Am. J. Cancer*, **15**, 2029–2043.

Shine, I. and Allison, P.R. (1966), Carcinoma of the oesophagus with tylosis (keratosis palmaris et plantaris). *Lancet*, **i**, 951–953.

Smith, R. and Gowing, N.F.C. (1953), Carcinoma of the oesophagus with histological appearances simulating a 'carcinosarcoma'. *Br. J. Surg.*, **40**, 487–489.

Staples, D.C., Knodell, R.G. and Johnson, L.F. (1978), Inflammatory pseudotumor of the esophagus. A complication of gastroesophageal reflux. *Gastrointest. Endosc.*, **24**, 175–176.

Stein, H.A., Murray, D. and Warner, H.A. (1981), Primary Hodgkin's disease of the esophagus. *Dig. Dis. Sci.*, **26**, 457–461.

Stern, Z., Sharon, P., Ligumsky, M. *et al.* (1980), Glycogenic acanthosis of the esophagus. A benign but confusing endoscopic lesion. *Am. J. Gastroenterol.*, **74**, 261–263.

Strauch, M., Martin, Th. and Remmele, W. (1971), Hodgkin's disease of the oesophagus. *Endoscopy*, **4**, 207–209.

Sweeney, E.C. and Cooney, T. (1980), Adenoid cystic carcinoma of the esophagus. A light and electron microscopic study. *Cancer*, **45**, 1516–1525.

Talbert, J.L. and Cantrell, J.R. (1963), Clinical and pathologic characteristics of carcinosarcoma of the esophagus. *J. Thorac. Cardiovasc. Surg.*, **45**, 1–12.

Tateishi, R., Taniguchi, H., Wada, A. *et al.* (1974), Argyrophil cell and melanocytes in esophageal mucosa. *Arch. Pathol.*, **98**, 87–89.

Tateishi, R., Taniguchi, K., Horai, T. *et al.* (1976), Argyrophil cell carcinoma (apudoma) of the esophagus. A histopathologic entity. *Virchows Arch. (Pathol. Anat.)*, **371**, 283–294.

Totten, R.S., Stout, A.P., Humphreys, G.H. II and Moore, R.L. (1953), Benign tumors and cysts of the esophagus. *J. Thorac. Surg.*, **25**, 606–622.

Turnbull, A.D., Rosen, P., Goodner, J.T. and Beattie, E.J. (1973), Primary malignant tumors of the esophagus other than typical epidermoid carcinoma. *Ann. Thorac. Surg.*, **15**, 463–473.

Voirol, M.W., Welsh, R.A. and Genet, E.F. (1973), Esophagitis cystica. *Am. J. Gastroenterol.*, **59**, 446–453.

Weitzner, S. (1970), Mucoepidermoid carcinoma of esophagus. Report of a case. *Arch. Pathol.*, **90**, 271–273.

Wynder, E.L., Hultberg, S., Jacobsson, F. and Bross, I.J. (1957), Environmental factors in cancer of the upper alimentary tract. A Swedish study with special reference to Plummer-Vinson (Paterson-Kelly) syndrome. *Cancer*, **10**, 470–487.

Zeabart, L.E., Fabian, J. and Nord, H.J. (1979), Squamous papilloma of the esophagus. A report of 3 cases. *Gastrointest. Endosc.*, **25**, 18–20.

5   The normal gastric mucosa

5.1   Endoscopic appearances

The mucosa of the stomach is smooth, glistening and appears yellow, orange, or red according to the brightness of the light source. The pylorus and cardia appear slightly paler than the body. Normally blood vessels cannot be recognized. On close inspection shallow grooves subdivide the mucosa into small, regular, slightly bulging areae gastricae. Parallel longitudinal gastric folds are largest and have a tortuous configuration adjacent to the greater curve and are smallest and most easily effaced by air insufflation along the lesser curve. The antral mucosa appears generally smooth although a few small longitudinal or circular folds can be present. A transverse fold, the angulus, is present at the antral-body junction.

5.2   Histology

Histologically the mucosa of the stomach can be divided into two layers – superficial and deep. Throughout the stomach the superficial zone is composed of a surface epithelium consisting of a single layer of tall, regular, mucin-secreting cells with basal nuclei, which dips down to form crypts (also termed pits or foveolae) lined by similar cells, although the amount of intracellular mucus decreases in the direction of the neck (or isthmus) of the glands. The deep layer consists of the glands which open into the bottom of the crypts. The composition of the glands varies and on the basis of their differing structure the gastric mucosa is divided into cardiac, body and pyloric types (see below).

Throughout the gastric mucosa the lamina propria consists of a network of collagen and reticulin fibres, more marked in the pylorus than the body region, with occasional fibroblasts, macrophages, eosinophils, plasma cells, mast cells and lymphocytes. The latter may be aggregated in the cardiac and pyloric regions to form small lymphoid follicles at the junction of the mucosa and submucosa, and less well defined aggregates of lymphocytes also occasionally occur in the body mucosa at this interface (Fig. 5.1).

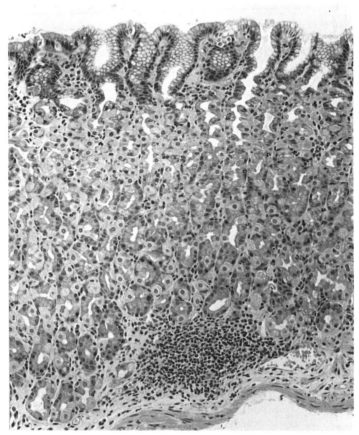

Fig. 5.1 Normal body mucosa. A small lymphoid aggregate is present. HE × 138.

5.2.1 Cardiac mucosa

This extends distally from its sharp junction with the stratified squamous epithelium of the oesophagus for a variable distance of 0.5 cm up to 3–4 cm. Because it straddles the anatomical boundary of the oesophagus and stomach it has also been referred to as junctional mucosa. Approximately half the mucosal thickness is occupied by pits. The underlying glands, which are simple tubular or compound tubulo-racemose in type, are lined by mucin-secreting cells, but occasional parietal and even chief cells can be present. Endocrine cells are frequent. The glands are often coiled and split up into groups or lobules by prolongations of the muscularis mucosae (Fig. 5.2). Cystic dilatation of the glands is common (Bensley, 1902).

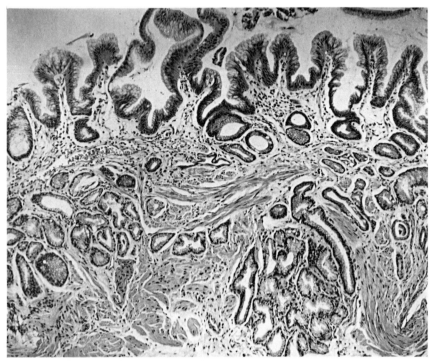

Fig. 5.2 Normal cardiac mucosa. Lobulated mucous glands with interdigitating smooth muscle fibres. HE × 90.

5.2.2 *Body mucosa*

The major part of the lining of the stomach consists of the body mucosa which under the dissecting microscope has a honeycomb (or Morocco leather) appearance with a regular pattern of closely packed papillae with a circular gastric pit opening at the apex of each (Salem and Truelove, 1964). Around groups of these papillae, each making up an area gastrica some 1–6 mm in diameter, are crevices formed by the fusion of pits occurring near the surface at a very acute angle. However, many pits open directly onto the surface and pit fusion is much less marked than in the pyloric mucosa (Goldstein *et al.*, 1969).

The body mucosa is from 400 to 1500 μm (0.4 to 1.5 mm) thick of which approximately a quarter is the superficial zone and the remainder the deeper glandular zone (Fig. 5.3). The glands consist of simple, straight, tightly packed tubules extending from the crypts to the muscularis mucosae where their blind ends are slightly thickened and coiled and may rarely be dilated. One to four glands open through a slight constriction or neck into the bottom of each crypt. The four types of cell present in the body glands are the mucous neck cells, parietal or oxyntic cells, chief or zymogenic cells and endocrine cells.

The mucin-secreting neck cells are relatively few in number and are scattered amongst the parietal cells at the junction of the glands with the pits, although they can occur deeper in the glands particularly near the pyloric region (Rubin *et al.*, 1968). They are fairly small, approximately 7 μm in width, with an irregular shape, appearing to be deformed by neighbouring cells, and with a basal nucleus and finely granular

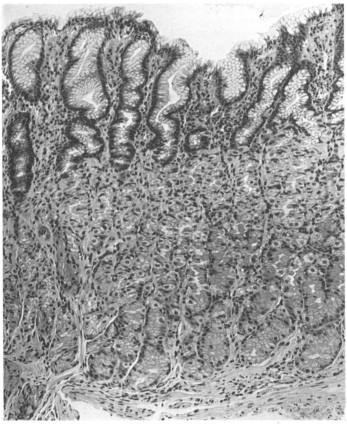

Fig. 5.3 Normal body mucosa. Short gastric pits with underlying tightly packed glands. HE × 132.

cytoplasm which stains positively with the periodic acid-Schiff reaction
although less than the surface and foveolar epithelial cells. Most of the
cells lining the upper part of the glands are parietal cells, the source of
hydrochloric acid, blood group substances and intrinsic factor. These are
large (20–35 μm), round or pyramidal cells with a central nucleus and an
eosinophilic vacuolated cytoplasm corresponding to the extensive
secretory canaliculus seen ultrastructurally. Their longest side is in
apposition to the basement membrane and their apical end wedged
between adjoining cells. Zymogen or chief cells, which secrete pepsinogen and other proteolytic pro-enzymes, predominate in the lower half of
the gland and intermingle with parietal cells in the middle third (Fig. 5.4).

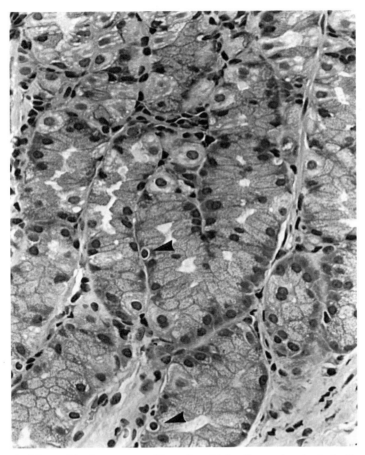

Fig. 5.4 Normal body mucosa. Granular chief cells predominate in the lower
part of the glands, parietal cells with central nuclei and perinuclear vacuolation in
the upper part. Note 'halo' endocrine cells (arrowed) HE × 375.

In freshly fixed material their cytoplasm contains refractile granules which are variably basophilic. They have a large basal nucleus. The numbers of chief and parietal cells in individual glands varies in different parts of the body of the stomach with a progressive increase in parietal cells and corresponding decrease in chief cells as the pyloric region is approached (Hogben *et al.*, 1974). Endocrine cells are described below (Section 5.2.5).

5.2.3 Pyloric mucosa

This occupies a roughly triangular area in the lower third of the stomach, with the boundary with body mucosa extending as an oblique line from a point about two-fifths of the way along the lesser curve to a point on the greater curve much nearer the pylorus. However, there is considerable individual variation especially in its extension along the lesser curve, so that it may reach almost to the cardia particularly in women (Landboe-Christensen, 1944; Oi *et al.*, 1959). With the dissecting microscope it has a coarser appearance than the body mucosa with a uniform mosaic pattern with several papillae in each segment (Salem and Truelove, 1964). The mucosa is from 200 to 1000 μm thick and the gastric pits are deeper and branch more than those in the body of the stomach. The glandular zone, composed of single or branched coiled tubules, surrounded at their bases by smooth muscle from the muscularis mucosae, occupies half or less of the total mucosal thickness (Fig. 5.5). The glands are less tightly packed than in the body mucosa and intertubular reticulin is increased. They are lined by faintly granular mucin-secreting cells with a basal nucleus and are indistinguishable from mucous neck cells in sections stained with haematoxylin and eosin. Occasional parietal cells are present in all parts of the pyloric mucosa and may be more numerous in biopsies close to the gastroduodenal junction (Tominaga, 1975). The most useful criteria for distinguishing body and pyloric mucosa in the normal stomach are the disappearance of chief cells from the latter (Grossman, 1960) and the change from single tubular glands in the body to branched glands in the antrum.

5.2.4 Transitional mucosa

The junction between the different types of gastric mucosa may be clear-cut or be occupied by a transitional type of mucosa in which the pits occupy half the mucosal thickness and the glandular zone consists of both body and pyloric or cardiac glands (Fig. 5.6).

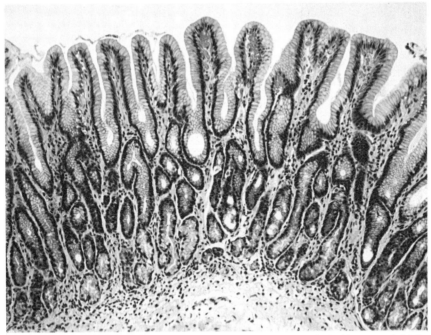

Fig. 5.5 Normal pyloric mucosa. Pits occupy approximately half mucosal thickness and show some branching. Underlying simple mucous glands. HE × 138.

5.2.5 Endocrine cells

These are widely and patchily distributed in the mucosa of all parts of the stomach (for good recent reviews see Lechago, 1978; O'Briain and Dayal, 1981). They may be recognized in haemotoxylin and eosin-stained preparations as rounded clear or halo cells in the glandular layer often wedged between the basement membrane of the glands and the epithelial cells (Fig. 5.4). In some cases red or pink granules are seen in an infranuclear position. A minority of these cells which contain serotonin (5–hydroxytryptamine), so-called enterochromaffin (EC) or argentaffin cells, may be demonstrated by their property of reducing silver salts without exposure to a reducing substance and by a positive diazo reaction. The majority of endocrine cells are argyrophilic with the Grimelius technique on formalin-fixed tissue. Some endocrine cells fail to stain with either argentaffin or argyrophil methods but may be demonstrated immunocytochemically. Recent work suggests that the enzyme neuron specific enolase is present in all currently identifiable endocrine cells (Fig. 5.7) and in the nerves of the gastrointestinal tract (Bishop *et al.*, 1982). Immunohistochemical staining techniques using

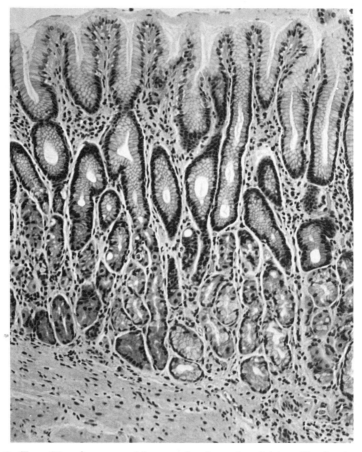

Fig. 5.6 Transitional mucosa. Mucous glands on the right and body glands on the left. HE × 174.

antibodies specifically directed against biogenic amines or polypeptide hormones have identified in the body and antrum of the stomach D cells which produce somatostatin, EC_n cells which contain serotonin, D_1 cells which are VIP (vasoactive intestinal peptide) immunoreactive cells, P cells containing bombesin, and PP cells (pancreatic polypeptide). Enterochromaffin-like (ECL) cells are confined to the body of the stomach and are the most common endocrine cell at this site, occurring in the inter-

Fig. 5.7 (a) Endocrine cells in the antrum immunostained for neuron specific enolase (NSE). PAP method × 450. (b) Adjacent 3 µm serial section immunostained for gastrin. The same cells are immunoreactive for both NSE and gastrin (arrows). PAP method × 450.

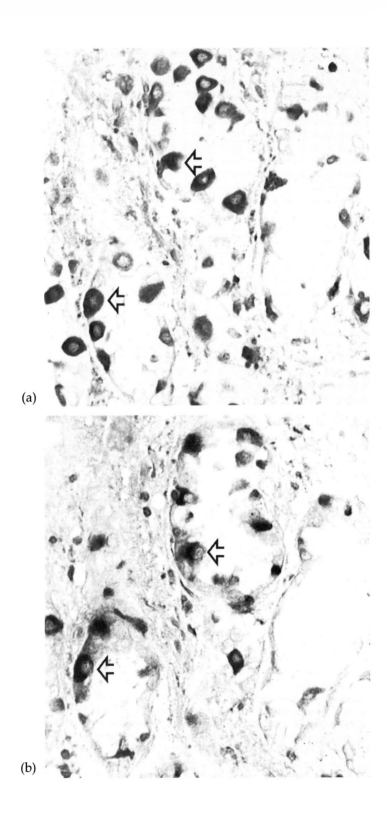

(a)

(b)

mediate and deep portions of the fundic glands. These cells have distinctive ultrastructural granules but no cell product has been identified. The same applies to so-called X cells which are Grimelius positive and occur principally in the oxyntic mucosa. S cells containing secretin have been identified in the lower third of the antropyloric mucosa. G cells are present predominantly in the lower and middle thirds of the antropyloric mucosa with relatively small numbers in the crypts and Brunner's glands of the proximal duodenum. They decrease in density from the pylorus to the gastric body (Voillemot *et al.*, 1978). They are the source of gastrin, the most investigated hormone of the gastrointestinal tract whose best-known function is its ability to stimulate gastric acid secretion. The cells are argyrophilic with the Grimelius technique and lead haematoxyphilic, and on ultrastructural examination contain rounded secretory granules with a variably electron-dense core and with an average diameter of 150–250 nm.

References

Bensley, R.R. (1902), The cardiac glands of mammals. *Am. J. Anat.*, **2**, 115–156.

Bishop, A.E., Polak, J.M., Facer, P. *et al.* (1982), Neuron specific enolase: a common marker for the endocrine cells and innervation of the gut and pancreas. *Gastroenterology*, **83**, 902–915.

Goldstein, A.M.B., Brothers, M.R. and Davis, E.A. Jr. (1969), The architecture of the superficial layer of the gastric mucosa. *J. Anat.*, **104**, 539–551.

Grossman, M.I. (1960), The pyloric gland area of the stomach. *Gastroenterology*, **38**, 1–6.

Hogben, C.A.M., Kent, T.H., Woodward, P.A. and Sill, A.J. (1974), Quantitative histology of the gastric mucosa: man, dog, cat, guinea pig, and frog. *Gastroenterology*, **67**, 1143–1154.

Landboe-Christensen, E. (1944), Extent of the pylorus zone in the human stomach. *Acta Pathol. Microbiol. Scand. (Suppl.)*, **54**, 671–692.

Lechago, J. (1978), Endocrine cells of the gastrointestinal tract and their pathology. In *Pathology Annual*, vol. 13, part 2 (ed. S.C. Sommers and P.P. Rosen), Appleton-Century-Crofts, New York, pp. 329–350.

O'Briain, D.S. and Dayal, Y. (1981), The pathology of the gastrointestinal endocrine cells. In *Diagnostic Immunocytochemistry* (ed. R.A. DeLellis), Masson, New York, pp. 75–109.

Oi, M., Oshida, K. and Sugimura, S. (1959), The location of gastric ulcer. *Gastroenterology*, **36**, 45–59.

Rubin, W., Ross, L.L., Sleisenger, M.H. and Jeffries, G.H. (1968), The normal human gastric epithelia. A fine structural study. *Lab. Invest.*, **19**, 598–626.

Salem, S.N. and Truelove, S.C. (1964), Dissecting microscope appearances of the gastric mucosa. *Br. Med. J.*, **ii**, 1503–1504.

Tominaga, K. (1975), Distribution of parietal cells in the antral mucosa of human stomachs. *Gastroenterology*, **69**, 1201–1207.

Voillemot, N., Potet, F., Mary, J.Y. and Lewin, M.J.M. (1978), Gastrin cell distribution in normal human stomachs and in patients with Zollinger-Ellison syndrome. *Gastroenterology*, **75**, 61–65.

6 Acute and chronic non-specific gastritis

'Gastritis is one of the most debated diseases. Its importance is often questioned. Some authors believe it to be one of the most important diseases of the human body; others deny its significance.' These sentiments by Schindler in the preface of his monograph on the subject (1947) are still applicable today and concern in particular the relationship of gastritis to the two most important conditions affecting the stomach, namely peptic ulcer disease and gastric cancer. In this chapter the histological features of acute and chronic gastritis will be described together with consideration of the pathogenesis and significance of chronic gastritis. Other types of gastritis are discussed in Chapter 7.

6.1 Acute gastritis

A variety of substances have been implicated in causing damage to the gastric mucosa including alcohol, aspirin, cortisone, phenylbutazone, indomethacin and a number of other non-steroidal anti-inflammatory drugs, although the evidence is largely circumstantial or anecdotal. In practice, acute gastritis is seen at endoscopy as a patchily or diffusely reddened mucosa, often with one or more erosions, in patients who have presented with haematemesis and/or melaena. A similar clinical picture can occur following trauma, sepsis, major surgery, burns or hypothermia. Haemorrhagic or erosive gastritis is common therefore in patients in intensive therapy units and in those with malignant disease (Klein *et al.*, 1973).

It is probable that aspirin interferes with the gastric mucosal 'barrier' by reducing the amount of mucus produced and altering its biochemical characteristics as well as inhibiting the local production of cytoprotective prostaglandins (Rees and Turnberg, 1980). Acid diffuses back into the mucosa with resultant histamine release and acute inflammation. In patients who are shocked and hypotensive, erosions probably develop on the basis of ischaemia due to a reduction in mucosal blood flow, again causing an increased permeability of the mucosa to hydrogen ions.

The distribution of erosions differs with the clinical circumstances. Following trauma or sepsis they are first observed in the fundus near the greater curve and with time develop distally, only involving the antrum when the lesions in the body are widespread and severe. This contrasts with erosions caused by aspirin and ethanol which, although most frequent in the antrum, can affect all segments of the stomach and the duodenum, and do not have a proximal to distal progression. The lesions also tend to be smaller and to heal quicker (Sugawa *et al.*, 1973; Metzger *et al.*, 1976; Hoftiezer *et al.*, 1982).

The indications for biopsy in these circumstances are few, mainly to exclude underlying disorders such as Crohn's disease, amyloidosis, Menetrier's disease and infiltrating carcinoma or lymphoma, where erosive changes may be conspicuous. Histologically there is oedema and haemorrhage into the interfoveolar subepithelial part of the lamina propria followed by necrosis of the surface epithelium and a variable amount of the underlying mucosa, with a surface slough consisting of degenerate epithelial cells, fibrin and some inflammatory cells (Figs 6.1 and 6.2). These different stages correspond to the red and white-based erosions seen endoscopically. Withdrawal of the initiating stimulus results in a rapid return of the mucosa to normal. It is unlikely that a single attack of haemorrhagic/erosive gastritis leads to chronic gastritis but repeated insults by agents such as alcohol and aspirin may do so. Some studies have shown that an antecedent chronic gastritis is often associated with haemorrhagic gastritis (Langman *et al.*, 1964; Winawer *et al.*, 1971). The relationship of aspirin to chronic gastric ulcer is discussed below (Section 6.2.2).

6.2   Chronic gastritis

Chronic non-specific gastritis is essentially a histological diagnosis and is the commonest change observed in biopsies from the stomach. There is a poor correlation between microscopical appearances and symptomatology. At endoscopy, gastritis may be recognized with reasonable accuracy (Myren and Serck-Hanssen, 1974), although its grading may not mirror the histological changes. As well as this approx-

---

Fig. 6.1   Gastric erosion. Intramucosal haemorrhage and focal disruption of surface epithelium. HE × 150.

Fig. 6.2   Gastric erosion. The superficial half of the mucosa consists of degenerate epithelial cells, fibrin and some inflammatory cells. There is haemorrhage beneath the surface epithelium in the intact mucosa. HE × 66.

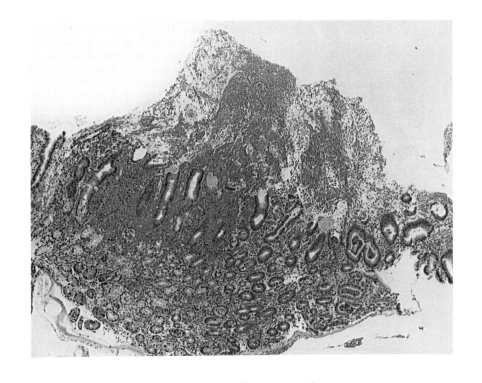

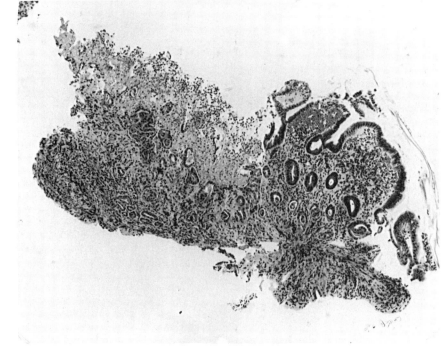

imately 30% of biopsies from endoscopically normal mucosa show inflammatory changes (Taor *et al.*, 1975). It is often patchy, and multiple biopsies may be necessary to diagnose and evaluate it. In addition individual biopsies have to be examined at different levels because of the frequently focal nature of the inflammation.

6.2.1 Classification

Classification of chronic non-specific gastritis (Whitehead *et al.*, 1972) takes into account (i) the type of mucosa i.e. cardiac, body, antral (pyloric), transitional or indeterminate, (ii) the extent of inflammation within the mucosa i.e. superficial or deep, the latter resulting in varying degrees of atrophy of the glandular compartment, (iii) the activity of the gastritis, and (iv) the presence and type of metaplasia. When this is done three histological patterns emerge, namely chronic superficial gastritis, atrophic gastritis, and gastric atrophy.

(a) *Chronic superficial gastritis.* As the name implies inflammation is confined to the superficial supraglandular layer of the mucosa (Figs 6.3 and 6.4). There is an increase in plasma cells and lymphocytes and sometimes eosinophils, together with variable numbers of polymorphs in

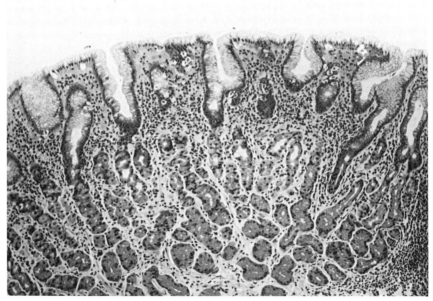

Fig. 6.3   Chronic superficial gastritis affecting body mucosa. HE × 105.

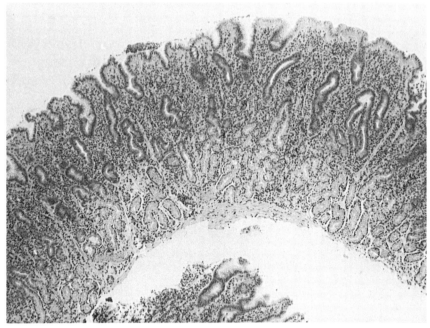

Fig. 6.4   Chronic superficial gastritis in antral mucosa. HE × 60.

the lamina propria between the foveolae and beneath the surface epithelium but not extending into the glandular layer. Although often focally distributed polymorphs are invariably seen and often extend into foveolar and surface epithelium. When active inflammation is marked the epithelium shows reactive changes with a cuboidal appearance of the cells associated with diminished cytoplasm and mucin content and enlargement and hyperchromatism of nuclei (Fig. 6.5). Marked regeneration of the surface epithelium can give a syncytial appearance with sprouting bud-like masses of cells, some of which appear to be in the process of exfoliation (Fig. 6.6). Collections of polymorphs may be seen in the pit lumens forming crypt abscesses, and moderate or severe acute inflammation can be associated with adhesion of surface and foveolar epithelial cells (Fig. 6.7). Oedema and vascular congestion may be a conspicuous feature. Foveolar hyperplasia results in the formation of intrafoveolar papillae giving a corkscrew appearance and a slight overall thickening of the mucosa (Fig. 6.8).

(b) *Atrophic gastritis.* In atrophic gastritis, inflammation involves the deeper layer of the mucosa and results in the destruction of the glands. The inflammatory cell content and its nature can be very variable. Minor

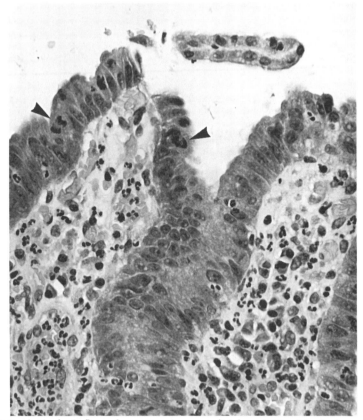

Fig. 6.5   Actively inflamed mucosa in superficial gastritis. Mucin has disappeared from the epithelial cells and polymorphs are prominent in the lamina propria and infiltrating the epithelium. Note mitoses (arrowed). HE × 375.

degrees of atrophy can be difficult to assess particularly in the pyloric mucosa and a stain for reticulin fibres to demonstrate their condensation around the glands can be helpful in this situation. In more advanced stages atrophy is readily apparent in routinely stained material as a widening and shortening of the glandular elements (Fig. 6.9). Accompanying this atrophic process two types of metaplasia occur, pseudo-pyloric and intestinal. The former involves only the body glands whose specialized cells are replaced by mucous cells derived from

Fig. 6.6   Syncytial groups of surface epithelial cells in actively inflamed gastric mucosa. HE × 159.

Fig. 6.7   Acutely inflamed gastric mucosa with crypt abscess to left and adhesion of epithelial cells across foveolae (arrowed). HE × 102.

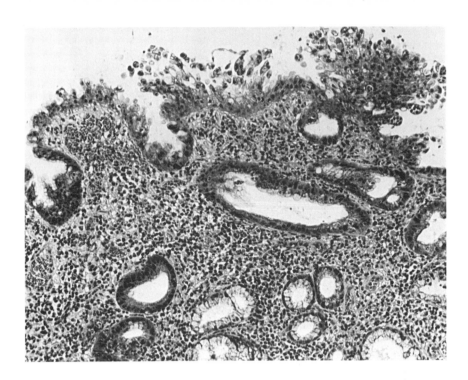

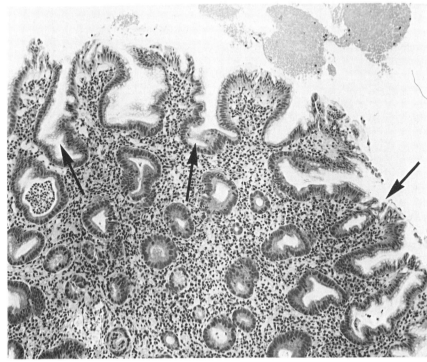

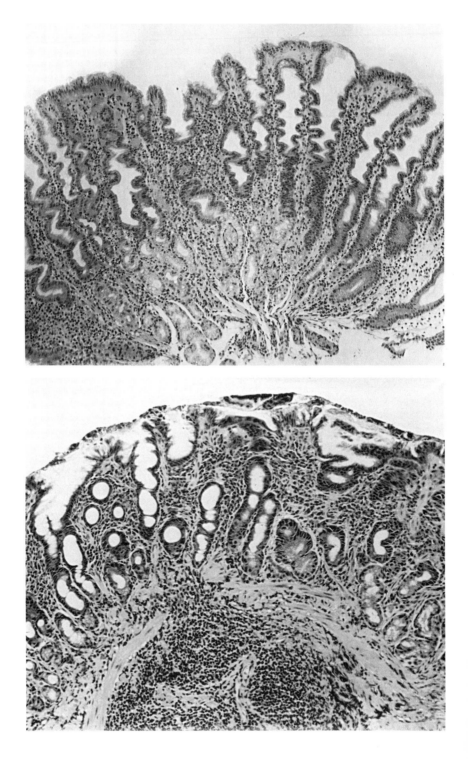

proliferated mucous neck cells and so initially affects the necks of these glands (Fig. 6.10). When widespread, the appearance of a biopsy from the body of the stomach may be indistinguishable from antral mucosa. However parietal cells are not seen, whereas they are frequently present in small numbers in the antral mucosa. As well as this gastrin cells are very scanty or absent in pseudo-pyloric metaplasia and common, although patchily distributed, in the antral mucosa (Sloan *et al.*, 1979).

Intestinal metaplasia is common in atrophic gastritis and can affect any part of the gastric mucosa, although most frequent in the antrum (Fig. 6.11). Oohara *et al.* (1983) observed it as a frequent change in the regenerative epithelium of gastric ulcers (Fig. 6.12). Its most characteristic feature is the presence of goblet cells which contain acidic mucins. These may be demonstrated with muci-carmine, or with the periodic acid –

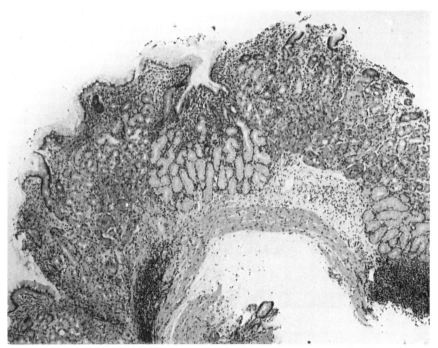

Fig. 6.10   Focal pseudo-pyloric metaplasia in gastric body mucosa. HE × 60.

Fig. 6.8.   Foveolar hyperplasia giving a corkscrew appearance in superficial antral gastritis. Interfoveolar adhesion of epithelial cells is a prominent feature. HE × 90.

Fig. 6.9   In this antral biopsy there is extension of inflammation into the glandular layer of the mucosa. Glands are separated and the mucosal thickness is reduced. HE × 126.

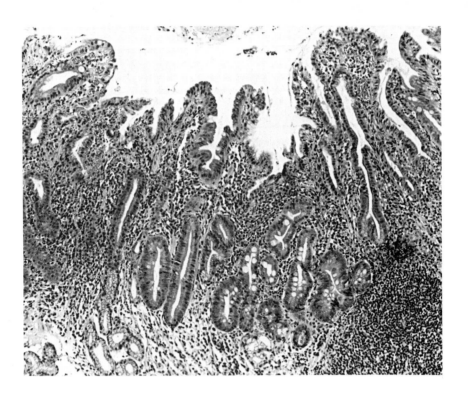

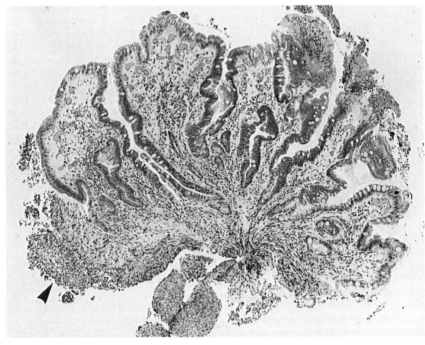

Schiff/alcian blue (PAS/AB) technique at pH 2.5 where they stain blue, in contrast to the PAS-positive neutral mucins present in surface and foveolar epithelium and the mucous glands of the non-metaplastic gastric mucosa. In its fully developed or complete form intestinal metaplasia consists of cells which are normally present in the small intestine. Goblet cells are separated by non-mucin secreting columnar cells which have a distinct striated border of microvilli. Goblet cells tend to be fewer in the deeper part of the mucosa (Fig. 6.13). At the base of the metaplastic

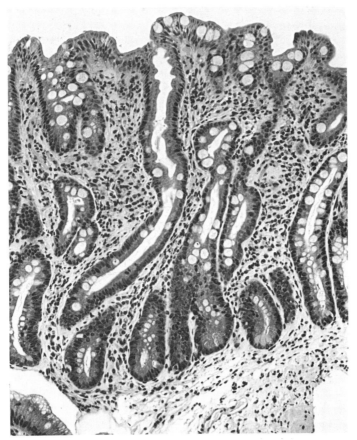

Fig. 6.13 Intestinal metaplasia (complete type). Goblet cells interspersed with columnar cells in which mucin is absent. HE × 150.

Fig. 6.11 An area of intestinal metaplasia in actively inflamed antral mucosa. Some residual pyloric glands are seen at lower left. HE × 102.

Fig. 6.12 Actively inflamed gastric mucosa with foveolar hyperplasia and intestinal metaplasia. Note ulcer slough (arrowed). HE × 60.

glands Paneth cells are present (Fig. 6.14) together with endocrine cells, many of which are argentaffin. Enzyme histochemistry and ultrastructural studies (Wattenberg, 1959; Lev, 1966) show similar features to small intestinal mucosa but a villous architecture is only rarely discernible (Fig. 6.15). In biopsies, foci of intestinal metaplastic epithelium may stain much darker than surrounding unaffected gastric epithelium and because of this may be misinterpreted as neoplastic (Fig. 6.16).

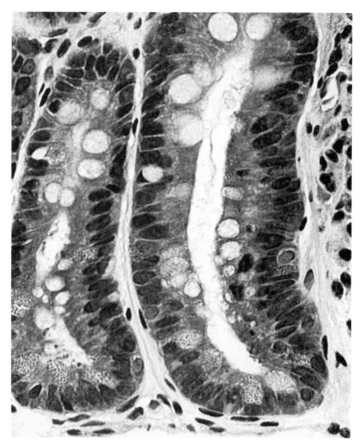

Fig. 6.14 Intestinal metaplasia (complete type). Paneth cells at crypt bases. HE × 600.

Fig. 6.15 This antral biopsy shows extensive intestinal metaplasia with only occasional groups of residual mucous glands. The surface has a low villous configuration. HE × 47.

Fig. 6.16 The darkly staining bases of metaplastic glands contrast with the surrounding pyloric glands. HE × 96.

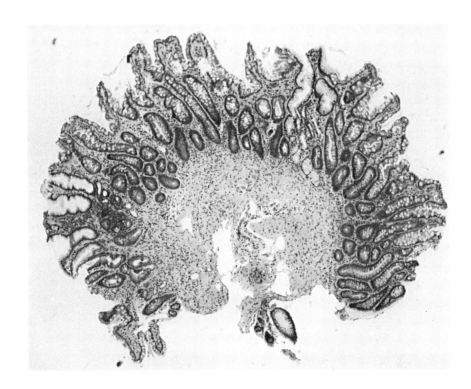

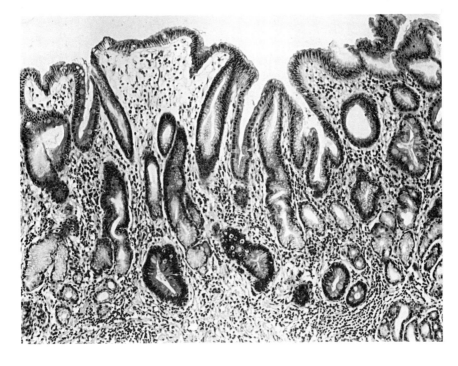

As well as this complete form, incomplete types of intestinal metaplasia are less commonly present (Ming *et al.*, 1967; Jass, 1980). In one of these a mixture of gastric and small intestinal epithelium is seen, with goblet cells interspersed with columnar cells which secrete predominantly neutral mucins. In another type, intervening columnar cells are distended with mucus and thereby often difficult to distinguish from goblet cells. However staining with high iron diamine/alcian blue (HID/AB) at pH 2.5 shows them to contain abundant sulphomucins, in contrast to the non-sulphated sialomucins usually present in the goblet cells (Fig. 6.17). In this respect therefore characteristics of colonic rather than small intestinal epithelium are present, although unlike the former no secretion of *O*-acylated sialic acid occurs (Jass, 1980; Segura and Montero, 1983). In both

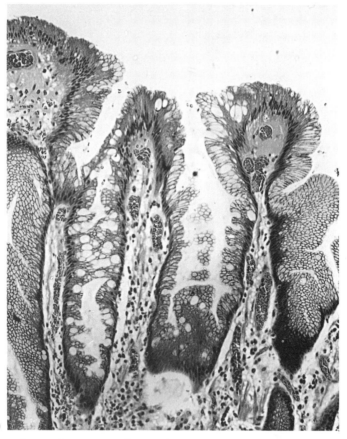

(a)

Fig. 6.17 Incomplete intestinal metaplasia. (a) Goblet cells are interspersed with tall columnar cells with apical mucin. HE × 150. (b) The mucin in the columnar

types of incomplete metaplasia Paneth cells are uncommon. Individual cells tend to be taller in incomplete compared with complete metaplasia and in the 'colonic' variant, elongation, tortuosity and branching of the metaplastic glands is prominent (Jass, 1980). There is indirect evidence that the type of intestinal metaplasia associated with sulphomucin secretion may be pre-malignant (Section 6.2.2).

Intestinal metaplasia can be focal or extensive and be quiescent or associated with active inflammation. The PAS/AB stain is very helpful in demonstrating its extent in biopsies. Morphological and autoradiographic studies indicate that intestinal metaplasia starts on the framework of an intact mucosa in the neck region of the gastric glands (Stemmermann and Hayashi, 1968; Hattori and Fujita, 1979). Thus in

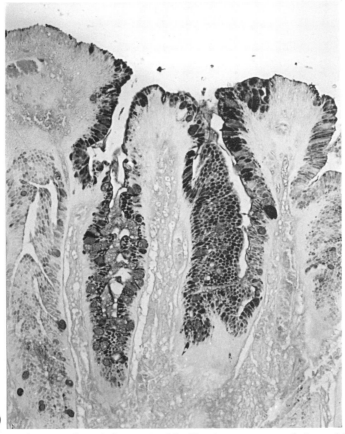

(b)

cells is predominantly sulphomucin (black) whereas most of the goblet cells secrete sialomucins (grey). HID/AB × 150.

antral biopsies it is not infrequent to see partially intestinalized glandular tubules, the upper parts of which are lined by intestinal cells and the lower parts by mucous gland cells (Fig. 6.18). The latter are replaced by intestinal epithelium and the generative zone shifts from the neck region to the base of one of the branched pyloric glands, with the disappearance of the other glands.

The mucosa in atrophic gastritis is in general thinner than normal although hyperplasia of the foveolar area can be marked. Sometimes however foci of intestinal metaplasia stand proud of the surrounding mucosa, resulting in a mamillated appearance when viewed at endoscopy. Mitotic counts reflect a high cell turnover in atrophic gastritis (Croft *et al.*, 1966). In some cases of superficial and atrophic gastritis hyperplasia of lymphoid tissue is conspicuous (Fig. 6.19) and occasionally cystic change can affect glands in either the antral or body mucosa. Slips of smooth muscle derived from the muscularis mucosae are often a prominent feature and may be particularly obvious in tangentially sectioned biopsies (Fig. 6.20).

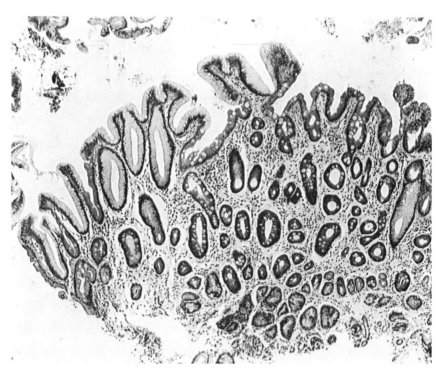

Fig. 6.18 Abrupt transition between mucin-secreting epithelium and epithelium which has undergone intestinal metaplasia. In some areas partially intestinalized glands are present. HE × 60.

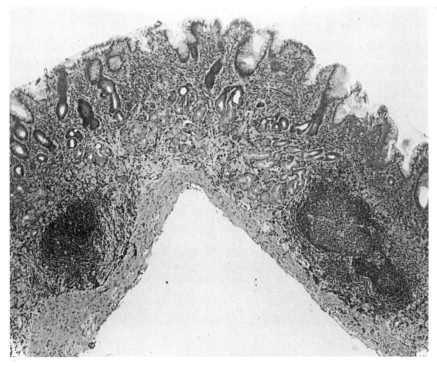

Fig. 6.19 Superficial gastritis in an antral biopsy associated with hyperplasia of lymphoid tissue. HE × 57.5.

(c) *Gastric atrophy.* In gastric atrophy the mucosa is markedly thinned with complete or near complete loss of glands and an absence of inflammation, although lymphoid aggregates can be present (Fig. 6.21). Tubules are lined by simple epithelium resembling surface epithelium and there is variable intestinal metaplasia. Fat spaces can be present in the prominent lamina propria and the muscularis mucosae is often markedly thickened.

6.2.2 Pathogenesis and significance of chronic gastritis

Chronic gastritis is a common disorder. In a recent study from Holland in which biopsies were taken from standardized sites in the stomach and duodenum atrophic gastritis involved the antrum alone in 6% and antral and body mucosa in a further 28% of asymptomatic volunteers whose average age was 33 years (Kreuning *et al.*, 1978). Epidemiological studies have shown variations in the prevalence of chronic gastritis. For example,

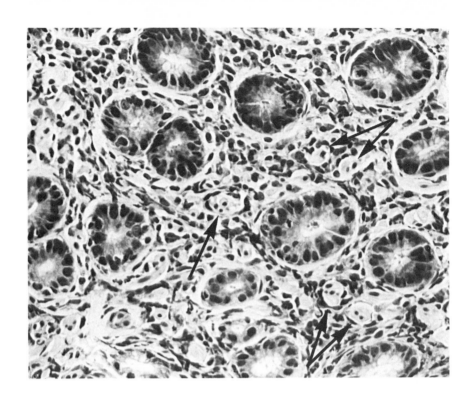

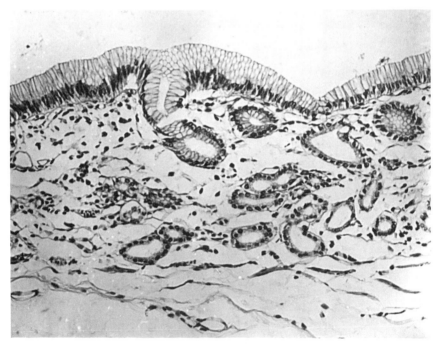

it was detected in 78% of Japanese over the age of 50 compared to 30% of Americans (Imai *et al.*, 1971). Follow-up studies within populations have shown an increasing prevalence of gastritis with age (Siurala *et al.*, 1968; Cheli *et al.*, 1973) which tends to progress from a superficial to an atrophic type, although this may be a very gradual process taking many years (Siurala *et al.*, 1968; Ormiston *et al.*, 1982). Based on differing clinical and pathological manifestations, two aetiologically distinct types of gastritis have been proposed (Strickland and Mackay, 1973).

In type A gastritis the body mucosa is predominantly affected with antral sparing. There is a high prevalence of antibodies to parietal cells (Taylor *et al.*, 1962), somewhat lower to intrinsic factor antibodies (Ardeman and Chanarin, 1966), and serum gastrin levels are usually elevated. The levels of pepsinogen I in the serum, which is derived only from body glands, are decreased, whereas those of pepsinogen II, which is produced by both fundic and pyloric gland cells, remain relatively normal (Samloff *et al.*, 1982). In a proportion of individuals with these features, overt or latent pernicious anaemia develops (Strickland and McKay, 1973). Clinical and serological evidence of associated autoimmune diseases such as Hashimoto's thyroiditis and adrenal Addison's disease is not uncommon (Doniach *et al.*, 1963). In first degree relatives of patients with pernicious anaemia, severe atrophic gastritis of the body mucosa, achlorhydria, parietal cell antibodies and a raised fasting serum gastrin level are considerably more common than in control subjects (Varis *et al.*, 1979), supporting the view that genetic factors are implicated in type A gastritis.

In type B gastritis, which is much commoner, the antrum is affected with or without body involvement, parietal cell antibodies are absent, serum gastrin levels are low, and acid secretion moderately to severely impaired. A variant of this type in which autoantibodies to gastrin-producing cells are present has recently been described (Vandelli *et al.*, 1979). Type B gastritis has been shown to spread proximally with increasing age, extending more rapidly on the lesser than on the greater curvature (Kimura, 1972). When the gastritis results in pseudo-pyloric metaplasia of body type mucosa the false impression is given of an expansion of the pyloric gland area (du Plessis, 1963). Endoscopic dye-spraying techniques using congo red to determine the extent of the acid-secreting area have shown that gastritis may also extend distally from the

---

Fig. 6.20   Individual and small groups of smooth muscle cells (arrowed) in the lamina propria. A common finding in gastritis. HE × 375.

Fig. 6.21   Gastric atrophy. Marked thinning of the mucosa and disappearance of specialized glandular cells is apparent in this biopsy of body mucosa. Inflammation is absent. HE × 195.

cardiac region of the stomach, again preferentially involving the lesser curve (Tatsuta *et al.*, 1974). The poor correlation of histological gastritis with symptoms, and the large number of ingested and endogenous agents which may theoretically damage the gastric mucosa has meant that no clear picture of the aetiology of this condition has emerged. Substances such as alcohol and salicylates, which are known to cause acute damage, might be expected to result in chronic gastritis when chronically administered but the evidence is conflicting. Parl *et al.* (1979) found a three times higher prevalence of chronic gastritis affecting the antrum of alcoholics over the age of 45 compared to non-alcoholics, whereas in another study patients with alcoholic and other types of cirrhosis showed a similar prevalence of chronic gastritis compared with age-matched controls (Brown *et al.*, 1981). There is a strong positive correlation between the heavy intake of aspirin and chronic gastric ulcer (Cameron, 1975; Piper *et al.*, 1981) but pathological examination of the stomach in many of these cases has shown an absence of chronic gastritis in the surrounding mucosa (Fig. 6.22). The ulcers are also unusual in that they are frequently located along the greater curvature (MacDonald, 1973; Hamilton and Yardley, 1980).

The role of duodenal reflux in the development of chronic gastritis and gastric ulceration was suggested by du Plessis (1960) who found an increased amount of bile acid conjugates in the fasting gastric aspirates of patients with gastric ulcers (1965). Regurgitation of duodenal contents into the stomach is much commoner in gastric ulcer patients than in healthy subjects or duodenal ulcer patients (Rhodes *et al.*, 1969). It is thought that bile acids probably acting with lysolecithin cause stripping of the surface mucus and depletion of mucus from the epithelial cells and at the same time allow hydrogen ions to diffuse back across the mucosa, initiating an inflammatory reaction subsequent to histamine release. Factors which are thought to predispose to reflux are poorly defined but probably include cigarette smoking (Taylor and Walker, 1980). It is also possible however that gastritis could be the initiating event in some cases.

The association of chronic gastritis with peptic ulceration of the stomach has long been recognized. Apart from pre-pyloric ulcers which share features with ulcers of the duodenum (Johnson, 1965), the majority of gastric ulcers occur on the lesser curve at the junction of antral and body type mucosa (Oi *et al.*, 1959). A minority arise entirely in the fundic mucosa (Tatsuta and Okuda, 1976). The higher up the lesser curve the ulcer is found, the more extensive the gastritis, with replacement of body glands by pyloric or intestinal metaplastic epithelium (Ball and James, 1961). High lying gastric ulcers heal more readily but are more prone to recurrence than more distal ulcers with less extensive gastritis (Tatsuta and Okuda, 1975). This, together with the fact that gastritis persists or

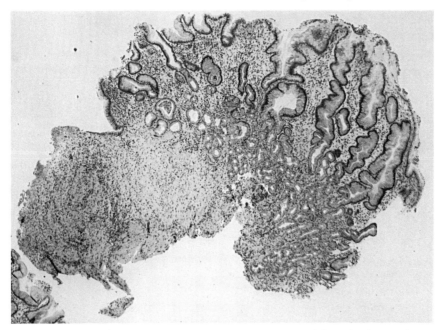

Fig. 6.22 Antral mucosa with minor inflammation and foveolar hyperplasia. Ulcer base to left. Biopsy from posterior wall ulcer adjacent to greater curve in chronic aspirin user. HE × 34.5.

worsens after ulcer healing (Mackay and Hislop, 1966; Gear *et al.*, 1971) suggests that ulcers arise on the basis of a preceding gastritis rather than that the inflammation is a secondary event following ulceration.

The relationship of chronic gastritis, and in particular intestinal metaplasia, to gastric cancer has been intensively studied. The prevalence of chronic atrophic gastritis is closely correlated with the death rate for gastric cancer in a population (Imai *et al.*, 1971) and follow-up studies have shown that it often precedes the development of gastric malignancy (Siurala *et al.*, 1966; Walker *et al.*, 1971). Intestinal metaplasia is commoner and more widespread in stomachs in which a cancer is present than in those with a benign lesion such as a peptic ulcer, and there is histological evidence that many gastric cancers arise from areas of intestinal metaplasia (Morson, 1955; Nakamura *et al.*, 1968), particularly those of intestinal type (Sipponen *et al.*, 1983). Studies in migrants moving from high incidence areas for gastric cancer have shown a reduction in the prevalence of intestinal metaplasia (Correa *et al.*, 1976; Stemmermann and Hayashi, 1968). Conflicting epidemiological data has come from a recent time trend study in Japan where a fall in prevalence of intestinal metaplasia appeared to follow a decline in the death rate from gastric cancer (Imai and Murayama, 1983). In populations at high risk for gastric cancer intestinal metaplasia is very common particularly at advanced ages, and in the United Kingdom (a population of intermediate risk) is seen in antral biopsies of some 20–30% of symptomatic individuals attending an endoscopy unit.

An assessment of the significance of the changes of chronic gastritis in an individual must take into account its distribution in the stomach (which means biopsies should be taken from several sites) and the age of the patient, along with clinical and functional data. These changes have to be correlated with those obtained in an age and sex-matched control population (Ihamaki *et al.*, 1979).

Because of the heterogeneous nature of intestinal metaplasia (Section 6.2.1) recent interest has focused on the significance and inter-relationships of the different variants. In several studies involving examination of resection specimens there has been a strong association between intestinal types of carcinoma and the presence in the adjacent mucosa of an incomplete type of metaplasia with prominent sulphomucin secretion (Heilmann and Hopker, 1979; Jass, 1980; Segura and Montero, 1983). This association was also present in an endoscopic biopsy study where, in all age groups, the prevalence and proportion of sulphomucin-positive intestinal metaplasia was higher in gastric cancer patients than in other groups (Sipponen *et al.*, 1980). The significance of this change as a more specific marker of pre-malignancy than intestinal metaplasia alone is currently being evaluated in long-term follow-up studies.

Two groups of patients who are known to be at increased risk of developing carcinoma are those with pernicious anaemia and individuals who have been operated on for benign peptic ulcer many years previously.

6.3 The stomach in pernicious anaemia

The main lesion in the stomach of patients with pernicious anaemia is an atrophic gastritis or gastric atrophy involving the body mucosa (Magnus, 1958). With gastritis there is a variable infiltrate of lymphocytes, plasma cells and eosinophils but neutrophils are often absent or few in number. Immunohistochemical investigation has shown an increase in both T and particularly B lymphocytes (Kaye *et al.*, 1982) and a reduction in the IgA/IgG ratio of immunoglobulin containing cells (Odgers and Wangel, 1968). Metaplasia of the body mucosa to small intestinal or more commonly pyloric type (Lewin *et al.*, 1976) is universal, although some residual, irregularly distributed parietal cells may be present. Both types of metaplasia can be seen together in biopsy material. The mucosa is usually markedly thinned (Fig. 6.23). However, a mamillated appearance of the fundic mucosa may be seen at endoscopy and biopsy of these small elevations shows hyperplastic areas of intestinal metaplasia. Biopsies from the antrum can be normal or show varying degrees of gastritis although this is often less than in the body. Antral gastritis is common in the general population and when present in patients with pernicious anaemia represents the coincidence of type A and type B gastritis in the same individual.

Quantitation of gastrin cells has shown increased numbers (Fig. 6.24) and a raised serum gastrin in those with a normal antral mucosa, but a marked reduction in both cell numbers and gastrin levels in the presence of antral atrophic gastritis (Stockbrugger *et al.*, 1977). Proliferation of endocrine cells in the body mucosa of the stomach and characterized as

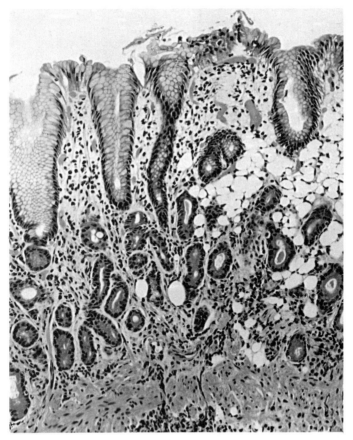

Fig. 6.23   Pernicious anaemia. Gastric body biopsy with thinning of the mucosa, loss of specialized glandular cells and fat spaces in the lamina propria. Appearances of gastric atrophy. HE × 150.

enterochromaffin-like (ECL) cells occurs in pernicious anaemia and other conditions with a raised serum gastrin (Section 8.1.2) and may occasionally result in single or multiple polypoid endocrine cell tumours (Figs 6.25 and 6.26). Other types of polyp have been observed at endoscopy in 20–37% of patients with pernicious anaemia (Elsborg *et al.*, 1977; Varis *et al.*, 1979; Stockbrugger *et al.*, 1983). They are mostly sessile, below 2 cm in diameter and frequently multiple. Histology has shown the majority to be hyperplastic in type, this often affecting particularly the foveolae, but some have shown dysplasia (Fig. 6.27). A recent biopsy study showed that dysplasia of moderate or severe degree was present in either the antrum or body in 11% of pernicious anaemia patients, and in the

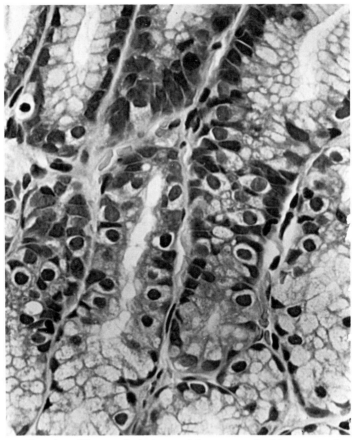

Fig. 6.24 Gastrin cell hyperplasia in pernicious anaemia. Numerous clear round cells with central nuclei in the mid-part of the antral glandular zone. Immunohistochemical staining demonstrated gastrin in these cells. HE × 600.

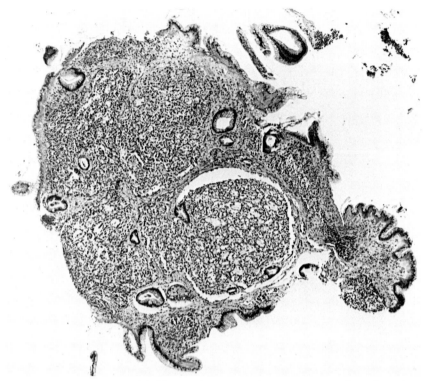

Fig. 6.25   Gastric carcinoid. Biopsy from one of numerous sessile polyps in a patient with pernicious anaemia. HE × 42.

majority the changes were diagnosed in samples taken from endoscopically visible lesions (Stockbrugger *et al.*, 1983).

The risk of cancer of the stomach in patients with pernicious anaemia appears to be at least three to four times that of the general population (Mosbech and Videbaek, 1950; Magnus, 1958). It is also of interest that a proportion of patients who present with gastric cancer without a previous history of pernicious anaemia have positive intrinsic factor antibodies and malabsorption of vitamin B_{12} reversed by administration of intrinsic factor, and appear therefore to be in a 'pre-pernicious anaemia stage' (Shearman *et al.*, 1966). The cancers in pernicious anaemia patients predominate in the fundic and cardiac areas of the stomach are often polypoid and commonly multiple (Schell *et al.*, 1954). It would appear justifiable to endoscope all patients in whom a diagnosis of pernicious anaemia is made. The indications for follow-up examinations and their frequency is currently being investigated.

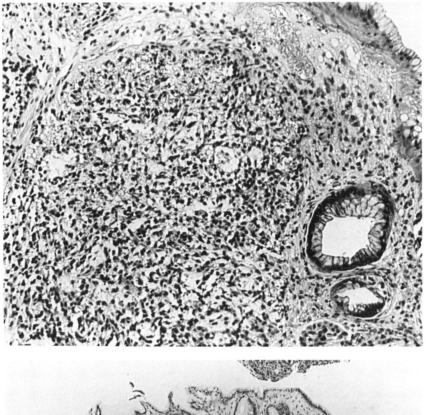

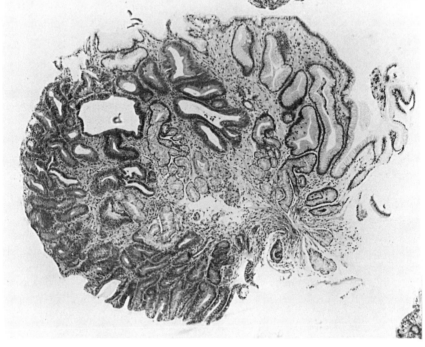

6.4   The operated stomach

Major importance is attached to the operated stomach as a precancerous condition and this will be considered below. However, a number of other changes may be observed at endoscopy or histologically following gastric surgery for benign disease, irrespective of whether or not a resection has been carried out. The commonest of these is atrophic gastritis which develops rapidly after operation and in one study was present in 54% of patients at two years, affecting 81% of those operated on for antral or pyloric canal ulcers (Pulimood *et al.*, 1976). At longer follow-up, gastritis is almost invariable. Atrophic changes are particularly marked in the gastric mucosa close to the stoma, whereas inflammation can be more conspicuous although often patchy in the remnant mucosa away from the anastomotic site (Saukonnen *et al.*, 1980). Loss of specialized cells is common and initially may selectively affect parietal cells (Fig. 6.28), with glands composed of chief and mucous cells only (Sipponen *et al.*, 1976). Gland irregularity and cyst formation is frequent, the cysts usually being lined by mucous cells, and pseudo-pyloric and intestinal metaplasia are very common. Slips of smooth muscle from the muscularis mucosae may extend between the glands. All these changes are more conspicuous close to the stoma and biopsies from this area are often characteristic (Figs 6.29 and 6.30).

Polyps occurring at or close to the stoma have been reported in about 10% of cases at long-term follow-up (Janunger and Domellöf, 1978; Savage and Jones, 1979). Macroscopically they may be single or multiple, discrete or confluent and occur along the line of anastomosis on the gastric side. Histologically they have usually been of hyperplastic or regenerative type and cystic change has been common. In a proportion of cases (Fig. 6.31) cysts lined by columnar or flattened mucous cells, but occasionally by parietal and chief cells, have been present in the submucosa, associated with irregularly arranged smooth muscle and collagen fibres (Littler and Gleibermann, 1972; Chakravorty and Schatzki, 1975; Stemmermann and Hayashi, 1979; Franzin and Novelli, 1981). The terms gastritis cystica polyposa (Littler and Gleibermann, 1972) and stomal polypoid hypertrophic gastritis (Koga *et al.*, 1979) have been used to describe this lesion, and its pathogenesis has been related to inflammation following biliary reflux, mucosal prolapse, ischaemia and the effects

---

Fig. 6.26   Detail of Fig. 6.25 shows uniform cells with pseudo-acinar arrangement. HE × 150.

Fig. 6.27   Gastric adenoma with moderate epithelial dysplasia. Sessile polyp at the antral-body junction. HE × 54.

of surgery including the presence of suture material (Griffel *et al.*, 1974; Franzin and Novelli, 1981).

The presence of lipid islands (xanthelasma) in the operated stomach is common (Fig. 6.32) and their prevalence increases with the length of follow-up (Section 13.4).

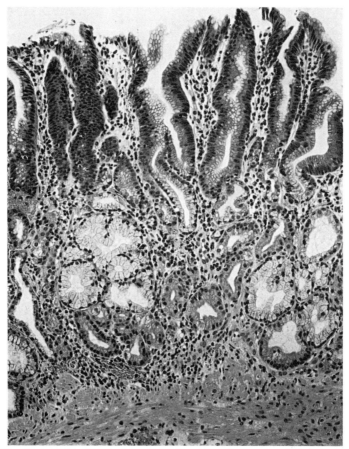

Fig. 6.28 Post-gastrectomy changes. Mucous cells occupy the upper parts of glands although deeper chief cells are preserved. Note foveolar hyperplasia. HE × 150.

Fig. 6.29 Post-gastrectomy changes. Pre-stomal biopsy in which there is inflammation, extensive pseudo-pyloric metaplasia and prominent glandular dilatation. HE × 67.

Fig. 6.30 Post-gastrectomy changes. Pseudo-pyloric metaplasia and cystic change in remnant stomach mucosa 20 years after Polya gastrectomy. Note marked foveolar hyperplasia. HE × 60.

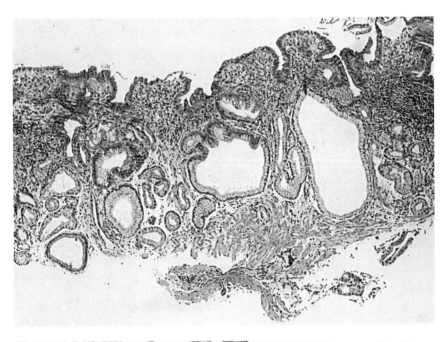

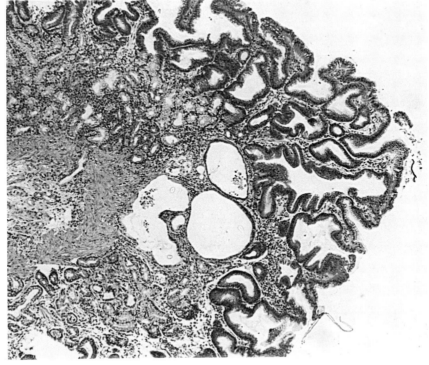

The relative risk of adenocarcinoma arising in the stomach of patients operated more than five years previously for benign conditions (more than 15 years previously for gastric malignancy) appears to be increased compared to the general population (Stalsberg and Taksdal, 1971; Domellof and Janunger, 1977; Corcoran *et al.*, 1984). The mean interval in most series between the time of operation and the diagnosis of malignancy has been from 20–30 years (Terjesen and Erichsen, 1976; Domellöf *et al.*, 1977; Schrumpf *et al.*, 1977), but with an inverse relation between age at operation and age at cancer manifestation (Giarelli *et al.*, 1983). No consistent difference in frequency has been found between patients operated on for gastric ulcer as compared with duodenal ulcer or relating to the type of operation carried out (Billroth I and Billroth II resection, gastrojejunostomy alone). The majority of cancers have occurred close to the site of anastomosis (Kobayashi *et al.*, 1970; Hammar, 1976; Domellöf *et al.*, 1977).

The diagnosis of carcinoma may only be made following histological examination of multiple biopsies since the endoscopic appearances may not suggest malignancy. Thus in one series only 28 (12%) of 226 biopsy specimens showed malignant or pre-malignant changes (Schrumpf *et al.*, 1977). As well as detecting carcinoma, some cases of which will be early

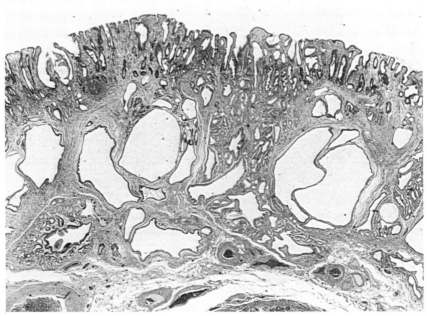

Fig. 6.31   Stomal polyp. Numerous submucosal cysts are present. HE × 15.

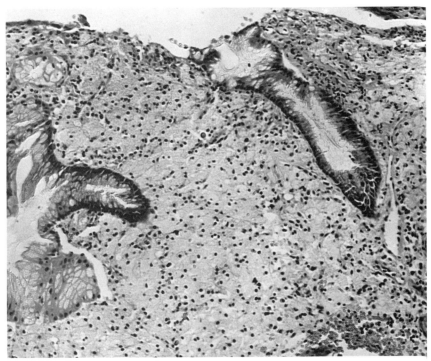

Fig. 6.32 Xanthelasma. Macrophages with foamy cytoplasm and small somewhat pyknotic nuclei fill the lamina propria. HE × 150.

gastric cancer (Osnes *et al.*, 1977), endoscopic examination of patients many years after gastric surgery has revealed epithelial changes of varying severity on biopsy which probably represent initial stages of gastric cancer, referred to as dysplasia (Section 9.1).

Minor epithelial changes of dysplasia merge into and are difficult to distinguish from regenerative or hyperplastic features (Figs 6.28 and 6.30), particularly when active inflammation is present. When these are excluded the proportion of patients showing dysplasia has varied from 7 to 21% in different series (Schrumpf *et al.*, 1977; Borchard *et al.*, 1979; Savage and Jones, 1979; Farrands *et al.*, 1983; Watt *et al.*, 1983). The prevalence of dysplasia may be related to a number of factors including the interval from operation, type of operation, number of biopsies taken and their site in the stomach and the variable cancer risks in the different geographical populations studied. As well as this a major factor is in the subjective assessment and interpretation of dysplasia (Section 9.1). Dysplasia can take the form of a focal sessile adenoma (Domellöf *et al.*, 1977; Borchard *et al.*, 1979), but more often has been described in a flat mucosa.

It may be widespread or multifocal and its detection has frequently been in asymptomatic individuals.

The finding of moderate or severe dysplasia in tissue samples merits close surveillance with repeat endoscopy and biopsy and consideration in the case of severe dysplasia of radical surgery. The role of screening in detecting gastric cancer in this group is contentious (Clémençon, 1979; Logan and Langman, 1983; Lund, 1983), but when individuals at risk do undergo endoscopy, for whatever reason, multiple biopsies should be taken particularly from the region of the stoma, together with cytological samples obtained by directed brushing.

References

Ardeman, S. and Chanarin, I. (1966), Intrinsic factor secretion in gastric atrophy. *Gut*, **7**, 99–101.

Ball, P.A.J. and James, A.H. (1961), The histological background to gastric ulcer. *Lancet*, **i**, 1365–1367.

Borchard, F., Mittelstaedt, A. and Kieker, R. (1979), Incidence of epithelial dysplasia after partial gastric resection. *Pathol. Res. Pract.*, **164**, 282–293.

Brown, R.C., Hardy, G.J., Temperley, J.M. *et al.* (1981), Gastritis and cirrhosis – no association. *J. Clin. Pathol.*, **34**, 744–748.

Cameron, A.J. (1975), Aspirin and gastric ulcer. *Mayo Clin. Proc.*, **50**, 565–570.

Chakravorty, R.C. and Schatzki, P.F. (1975), Gastric cystic polyposis. *Dig. Dis.*, **20**, 981–989.

Cheli, R., Santi, L., Ciancamerla, G. and Canciani, G. (1973), A clinical and statistical follow-up study of atrophic gastritis. *Dig. Dis.*, **18**, 1061–1066.

Clémençon, G. (1979), Risk of carcinoma in the gastric remnant after gastric resection for benign conditions. In *Gastric Cancer* (ed. Ch. Herfarth and P. Schlag), Springer-Verlag, Berlin, pp. 129–136.

Corcoran, G., Ware, J., Day, D. and Baxter, J.N. (1984), Gastric cancer developing after operations for benign peptic ulcer. *Gut*, **25**, 1183–1184 (abstract).

Correa, P., Cuello, C., Duque, E. *et al.* (1976), Gastric cancer in Colombia. III. Natural history of precursor lesions. *J. Natl. Cancer Inst.*, **57**, 1027–1035.

Croft, D.N., Pollock, D.J. and Coghill, N.F. (1966), Cell loss from human gastric mucosa measured by the estimation of desoxyribonucleic acid (DNA) in gastric washings. *Gut*, **7**, 333–343.

Domellöf, L. and Janunger, K-G. (1977), The risk for gastric carcinoma after partial gastrectomy. *Am. J. Surg.*, **134**, 581–584.

Domellöf, L., Eriksson, S. and Janunger, K-G (1977), Carcinoma and possible precancerous changes of the gastric stump after Billroth II resection. *Gastroenterology*, **73**, 462–468.

Doniach, D., Roitt, I.M. and Taylor, K.B. (1963), Autoimmune phenomena in pernicious anaemia: serological overlap with thyroiditis, thyrotoxicosis and systemic lupus erythematosus. *Br. Med. J.*, **i**, 1374–1379.

du Plessis, D.J. (1960), Some aspects of the pathogenesis and surgical management of peptic ulcers. *S. Afr. Med. J.*, **34**, 101–108.

du Plessis, D.J. (1963), The importance of the pyloric antrum in peptic ulceration. *S. Afr. J. Surg.*, **1**, 3–11.

du Plessis, D.J. (1965), Pathogenesis of gastric ulceration. *Lancet*, **i**, 974–978.

Elsborg, L., Andersen, D., Myhre-Jensen, O. and Bastrup-Madsen, P. (1977), Gastric mucosal polyps in pernicious anaemia. *Scand. J. Gastroenterol.*, **12**, 49–52.

Farrands, P.A., Blake, J.R.S., Ansell, I.D. *et al.* (1983), Endoscopic review of patients who have had gastric surgery. *Br. Med. J.*, **286**, 755–758.

Franzin, G. and Novelli, P. (1981), Gastritis cystica profunda. *Histopathology*, **5**, 535–547.

Gear, M.W.L., Truelove, S.C. and Whitehead, R. (1971), Gastric ulcer and gastritis. *Gut*, **12**, 639–645.

Giarelli, L., Melato, M., Stanta, G. *et al.* (1983), Gastric resection. A cause of high frequency of gastric carcinoma. *Cancer*, **52**, 1113–1116.

Griffel, B., Engleberg, M. and Reiss, R. (1974), Multiple polypoid cystic gastritis in old gastroenteric stoma. *Arch. Pathol.*, **97**, 316–318.

Hamilton, S.R. and Yardley, J.H. (1980), Endoscopic biopsy diagnosis of aspirin-associated chronic gastric ulcers. *Gastroenterology*, **78**, 1178 (abstract).

Hammar, E. (1976), The localization of precancerous changes and carcinoma after previous gastric operation for benign condition. *Acta Pathol. Microbiol. Scand.*, **84**, 495–507.

Hattori, T. and Fujita, S. (1979), Tritiated thymidine autoradiographic study on histogenesis and spreading of intestinal metaplasia in human stomach. *Pathol. Res. Pract.*, **164**, 224–237.

Heilmann, K.L. and Höpker, W.W. (1979), Loss of differentiation in intestinal metaplasia in cancerous stomachs. A comparative morphologic study. *Pathol. Res. Pract.*, **164**, 249–258.

Hoftiezer, J.W., O'Laughlin, J.C. and Ivey, K.J. (1982), Effects of 24 hours of aspirin, bufferin, paracetamol and placebo on normal human gastroduodenal mucosa. *Gut*, **23**, 692–697.

Ihamäki, T., Varis, K. and Siurala, M. (1979), Morphological, functional and immunological state of the gastric mucosa in gastric carcinoma families. Comparison with a computer-matched family sample. *Scand. J. Gastroenterol.*, **14**, 801–812.

Imai, T., Kubo, T. and Watanabe, H. (1971), Chronic gastritis in Japanese with reference to high incidence of gastric carcinoma. *J. Natl. Cancer Inst.*, **47**, 179–195.

Imai, T. and Murayama, H. (1983), Time trend in the prevalence of intestinal metaplasia in Japan. *Cancer*, **52**, 353–361.

Janunger, K-G. and Domellöf, L. (1978), Gastric polyps and precancerous mucosal changes after partial gastrectomy. *Acta Chir. Scand.*, **144**, 293–298.

Jass, J.R. (1980), Role of intestinal metaplasia in the histogenesis of gastric carcinoma. *J. Clin. Pathol.*, **33**, 801–810.

Johnson, H.D. (1965), Gastric ulcer: classification, blood group characteristics, secretion patterns and pathogenesis. *Ann. Surg.*, **162**, 996–1004.

Kaye, M.D., Whorwell, P.J. and Wright, R. (1982), Gastric mucosal lymphocyte populations in pernicious anemia (PA). *Gastroenterology*, **82**, 1097 (abstract).

Kimura, K. (1972), Chronological transition of the fundic–pyloric border determined by stepwise biopsy of the lesser and greater curvatures of the stomach. *Gastroenterology*, **63**, 584–592.

Klein, M.S., Ennis, F., Sherlock, P. and Winawer, S.J. (1973), Stress erosions. A major cause of gastrointestinal hemorrhage in patients with malignant disease. *Dig. Dis.*, **18**, 167–173.

Kobayashi, S., Prolla, J.C. and Kirsner, J.B. (1970), Late gastric carcinoma developing after surgery for benign conditions. Endoscopic and histologic studies of the anastomosis and diagnostic problems. *Dig. Dis.*, **15**, 905–912.

Koga, S., Watanabe, H. and Enjoji, M. (1979), Stomal polypoid hypertrophic gastritis. A polypoid gastric lesion at gastroenterostomy site. *Cancer*, **43**, 647–657.

Kreuning, J., Bosman, F.T., Kuiper, G. *et al.* (1978), Gastric and duodenal mucosa in 'healthy' individuals. An endoscopic and histopathological study of 50 volunteers. *J. Clin. Pathol.*, **31**, 69–77.

Langman, M.J.S., Hansky, J.H., Drury, R.A.B. and Jones, F.A. (1964), The gastric mucosa in radiologically negative acute gastrointestinal bleeding. *Gut*, **5**, 550–552.

Lev, R. (1966), The mucin histochemistry of normal and neoplastic gastric mucosa. *Lab. Invest.*, **14**, 2080–2100.

Lewin, K.J., Dowling, F., Wright, J.P. and Taylor, K.B. (1976), Gastric morphology and serum gastrin levels in pernicious anaemia. *Gut*, **17**, 551–560.

Littler, E.R. and Gleibermann, E. (1972), Gastritis cystica polyposa. (Gastric mucosal prolapse at gastroenterostomy site, with cystic and infiltrative epithelial hyperplasia.) *Cancer*, **29**, 205–209.

Logan, R.F.A. and Langman, M.J.S. (1983), Screening for gastric cancer after gastric surgery. *Lancet*, **ii**, 667–670.

Lund, E. (1983), Gastric cancer after gastric surgery: an increasing problem in Norway. *Lancet*, **ii**, 973 (letter).

MacDonald, W.C. (1973), Correlation of mucosal histology and aspirin intake in chronic gastric ulcer. *Gastroenterology*, **65**, 381–389.

MacKay, I.R. and Hislop, I.G. (1966), Chronic gastritis and gastric ulcer. *Gut*, **7**, 228–233.

Magnus, H.A. (1958), A re-assessment of the gastric lesion in pernicious anaemia. *J. Clin. Pathol.*, **11**, 289–295.

Metzger, W.H., McAdam, L., Bluestone, R. and Guth, P.H. (1976), Acute gastric mucosal injury during continuous or interrupted aspirin ingestion in humans. *Dig. Dis.*, **21**, 963–968.

Ming, S-C., Goldman, H. and Freiman, D.G. (1967), Intestinal metaplasia and histogenesis of carcinoma in human stomach. Light and electron microscopic study. *Cancer*, **20**, 1418–1429.

Morson, B.C. (1955), Carcinoma arising from areas of intestinal metaplasia in the gastric mucosa. *Br. J. Cancer*, **9**, 377–385.

Mosbech, J. and Videbaek, A. (1950), Mortality from and risk of gastric carcinoma among patients with pernicious anaemia. *Br. Med. J.*, **2**, 390–394.

Myren, J. and Serck-Hanssen, A. (1974), The gastroscopic diagnosis of gastritis. With particular reference to mucosal reddening and mucus covering. *Scand. J. Gastroenterol.*, **9**, 457–462.

Nakamura, K., Sugano, H. and Takagi, K. (1968), Carcinoma of the stomach in incipient phase: its histogenesis and histological appearances. *Gann*, **59**, 251–258.

Odgers, R.J. and Wangel, A.G. (1968), Abnormalities in IgA-containing mononuclear cells in the gastric lesion of pernicious anaemia. *Lancet*, **ii**, 846–849.

Oi, M., Oshida, K. and Sugimura, S. (1959), The location of gastric ulcer. *Gastroenterology*, **36**, 45–56.

Oohara, T., Tohma, H., Aono, G. *et al.* (1983), Intestinal metaplasia of the regenerative epithelia in 549 gastric ulcers. *Hum. Pathol.*, **14**, 1066–1071.

Ormiston, M.C., Gear, M.W.L. and Codling, B.W. (1982), Five year follow-up study of gastritis. *J. Clin. Pathol.*, **35**, 757–760.

Osnes, M. Lotveit, T., Myren, J. and Serck-Hanssen, A. (1977), Early gastric carcinoma in patients with a Billroth II partial gastrectomy. *Endoscopy*, **9**, 45–49.

Parl, F.F., Lev, R., Thomas, E. and Pitchumoni, C.S. (1979), Histologic and morphometric study of chronic gastritis in alcoholic patients. *Hum. Pathol.*, **10**, 45–56.

Piper, D.W., McIntosh, J.H., Ariotti, D.E. (1981), Analgesic ingestion and chronic peptic ulcer. *Gastroenterology*, **80**, 427–432.

Pulimood, B.M., Knudsen, A. and Coghill, N.F. (1976), Gastric mucosa after partial gastrectomy. *Gut*, **17**, 463–470.

Rees, W.D.W. and Turnberg, L.A. (1980), Reappraisal of the effect of aspirin on the stomach. *Lancet*, **ii**, 410–413.

Rhodes, J., Barnardo, D.E., Phillips, S.F. *et al.* (1969), Increased reflux of bile into the stomach in patients with gastric ulcer. *Gastroenterology*, **57**, 241–252.

Samloff, I.M., Varis, K., Ihamäki, T. *et al.* (1982), Relationships among serum pepsinogen I, serum pepsinogen II, and gastric mucosal histology. A study in relatives of patients with pernicious anemia. *Gastroenterology*, **83**, 204–209.

Saukkonen, M., Sipponen, P., Varis, K. and Siurala, M. (1980), Morphological and dynamic behavior of the gastric mucosa after partial gastrectomy with special reference to the gastroenterostomy area. *Hepato-Gastroenterol.*, **27**, 48–56.

Savage, A. and Jones, S. (1979), Histological appearances of the gastric mucosa 15–27 years after partial gastrectomy. *J. Clin. Pathol.*, **32**, 179–186.

Schell, R.F., Dockerty, M.B. and Comfort, M.W. (1954), Carcinoma of the stomach associated with pernicious anemia: a clinical and pathologic study. *Surg. Gynecol. Obstet.*, **98**, 710–720.

Schindler, R. (1947), *Gastritis*. William Heinemann, London.

Schrumpf, E., Serck-Hanssen, A., Stadaas, J. *et al.* (1977), Mucosal changes in the gastric stump 20–25 years after partial gastrectomy. *Lancet*, **ii**, 467–469.

Segura, D.I. and Montero, C. (1983), Histochemical characterization of different types of intestinal metaplasia in gastric mucosa. *Cancer*, **52**, 498–503.

Shearman D.J.C., Finlayson, N.D.C., Wilson, R. and Samson, R.R. (1966), Carcinoma of the stomach and early pernicious anaemia. *Lancet*, **ii**, 403–404.

Sipponen, P., Hakkiluoto, A., Kalima, T.V. and Siurala, M. (1976), Selective loss of parietal cells in the gastric remnant following antral resection. *Scand. J. Gastroenterol.*, **11**, 813–816.

Sipponen, P., Kekki, M. and Siurala, M. (1983), Atrophic chronic gastritis and intestinal metaplasia in gastric carcinoma. Comparison with a representative population sample. *Cancer*, **52**, 1062–1068.

Sipponen, P., Seppälä, K., Varis, K. *et al.* (1980), Intestinal metaplasia with colonic-type sulphomucins in the gastric mucosa; its association with gastric carcinoma. *Acta Pathol. Microbiol. Scand.*, *[A]*, **88**, 217–224.

Siurala, M., Varis, K. and Wiljasalo, M. (1966), Studies of patients with atrophic gastritis: a 10–15 year follow-up. *Scand. J. Gastroenterol.*, **1**, 40–48.

Siurala, M., Isokoski, M., Varis, K. and Kekki, M. (1968), Prevalence of gastritis in a rural population. Bioptic study of subjects selected at random. *Scand. J. Gastroenterol.*, **3**, 211–223.

Sloan, J.M., Buchanan, K.D., McFarland, R.J. *et al.* (1979), A histological study of the effect of chronic gastritis on gastrin cell distribution in the human stomach. *J. Clin. Pathol.*, **32**, 201–207.

Stalsberg, H. and Taksdal, S. (1971), Stomach cancer following gastric surgery for benign conditions. *Lancet*, **ii**, 1175–1177.

Stemmermann, G.N. and Hayashi, T. (1968), Intestinal metaplasia of the gastric mucosa: a gross and microscopic study of its distribution in various disease states. *J. Natl. Cancer Inst.*, **41**, 627–634.

Stemmermann, G.N. and Hayashi, T. (1979), Hyperplastic polyps of the gastric mucosa adjacent to gastroenterostomy stomas. *Am. J. Clin. Pathol.*, **71**, 341–345.

Stockbrügger, R., Larsson, L-T., Lundqvist, G. and Angervall, L. (1977), Antral gastrin cells and serum gastrin in achlorhydria. *Scand. J. Gastroenterol.*, **12**, 209–213.

Stockbrügger, R.W., Menon, G.G., Beilby, J.O.W. *et al.* (1983), Gastroscopic screening in 80 patients with pernicious anaemia. *Gut*, **24**, 1141–1147.

Strickland, R.G. and Mackay, I.R. (1973), A reappraisal of the nature and significance of chronic atrophic gastritis. *Dig. Dis.*, **18**, 426–440.

Sugawa, C., Lucas, C.E., Rosenberg, B.F. *et al.* (1973), Differential topography of acute erosive gastritis due to trauma or sepsis, ethanol and aspirin. *Gastrointest. Endosc.*, **19**, 127–130.

Taor, R.E., Fox, B., Ware, J. and Johnson, A.G. (1975), Gastritis – gastroscopic and microscopic. *Endoscopy*, **7**, 209–215.

Tatsuta, M. and Okuda, S. (1975), Location, healing, and recurrence of gastric ulcers in relation to fundal gastritis. *Gastroenterology*, **69**, 897–902.

Tatsuta, M. and Okuda, S. (1976), Gastric ulcers in the fundic gland area. *Gastroenterology*, **71**, 16–18.

Tatsuta, M., Saegusa, T. and Okuda, S. (1974), Extension of fundal gastritis studied by endoscopic congo red test. *Endoscopy*, **6**, 20–26.

Taylor, K.B., Roitt, I.M., Doniach, D. *et al.* (1962), Autoimmune phenomena in pernicious anaemia: gastric antibodies. *Br. Med. J.*, **2**, 1347–1352.

Taylor, W.H. and Walker, V. (1980), Smoking and peptic ulceration. *J. Roy. Soc. Med.*, **73**, 159–161.

Terjesen, T. and Erichsen, H.G. (1976), Carcinoma of the gastric stump after operation for benign gastroduodenal ulcer. *Acta Chir. Scand.*, **142**, 256–260.

Vandelli, C., Bottazzo, G.F., Doniach, D. and Franceschi, F. (1979), Autoantibodies to gastrin-producing cells in antral (type B) chronic gastritis. *N. Engl. J. Med.*, **300**, 1406–1410.

Varis, K., Ihamäki, T., Härkönen, M. *et al.* (1979), Gastric morphology, function, and immunology in first-degree relatives of probands with pernicious anemia and controls. *Scand. J. Gastroenterol.*, **14**, 129–139.

Walker, I.R., Strickland, R.G., Ungar, B. and Mackay, I.R. (1971), Simple atrophic gastritis and gastric carcinoma. *Gut*, **12**, 906–911.

Watt, P.C.H., Sloan, J.M. and Kennedy, T.L. (1983), Changes in gastric mucosa after vagotomy and gastrojejunostomy for duodenal ulcer. *Br. Med. J.*, **287**, 1407–1410.

Wattenberg, L.W. (1959), Histochemical study of aminopeptidase in metaplasia and carcinoma of the stomach. *Arch. Pathol.*, **67**, 281–286.

Whitehead, R., Truelove, S.C. and Gear, M.W.L. (1972), The histological diagnosis of chronic gastritis in fibreoptic gastroscope biopsy specimens. *J. Clin. Pathol.*, **25**, 1–11.

Winawer, S.J., Bejar, J., McCray, R.S. and Zamcheck, N. (1971), Haemorrhagic gastritis: importance of associated chronic gastritis. *Arch. Intern. Med.*, **127**, 129–131.

7 Other types of gastritis

7.1 Phlegmonous gastritis

Phlegmonous gastritis is a rare disease with a high mortality. Patients usually present with symptoms of severe epigastric pain often following systemic or localized infection elsewhere, particularly due to haemolytic streptococci. Chronic alcoholism has been a predisposing factor in some (Miller *et al.*, 1975) but it has also affected young previously healthy individuals (Bron *et al.*, 1977). The stomach is dilated and giant purple mucosal folds with a spongy consistency are seen at endoscopy. The main changes are in the submucosa and may be demonstrated in a snare biopsy. There is marked purulent inflammation and oedema, and thrombosis of blood vessels.

7.2 Varioliform (verrucous) gastritis

This condition has a characteristic endoscopic and radiological appearance. There are multiple small raised nodules with a central necrotic area which are typically longitudinally arranged along folds of the greater curvature, and anterior and posterior walls of the antrum. Sometimes they have occurred in the fundus and cardiac regions. The occasional large, single lesions may resemble an early gastric cancer at endoscopy. Individual lesions have been termed complete erosions (Roesch, 1978) or aphthous ulcers (Morgan *et al.*, 1976). Histologically there is an erosive defect associated with a fibrinopurulent exudate. There can be marked regenerative changes in the underlying and adjacent mucosa with sheets of closely packed, variably distorted glands with swollen lining cells and hyperchromatic nuclei. These are set in an amorphous eosinophilic background matrix (Figs. 7.1 and 7.2). This appearance may be misinterpreted as malignant (Isaacson, 1982), but mitoses are not a prominent feature and there is a gradual transition to more obviously benign regenerating mucosa at the margin of the erosion

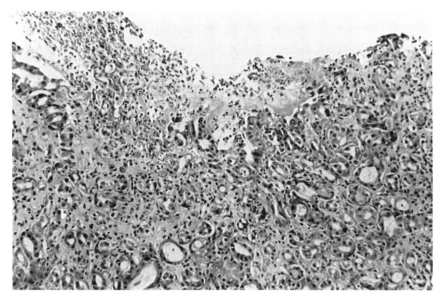

Fig. 7.1 Varioliform gastritis. Erosion of the surface epithelium with disorganized underlying glands merging into normal appearing glands (right). HE × 100.

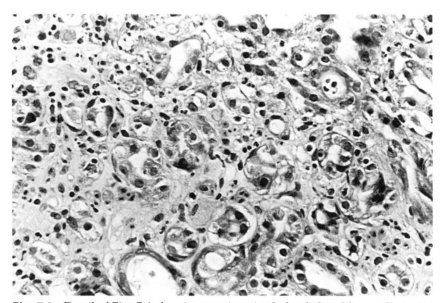

Fig. 7.2 Detail of Fig. 7.1 showing varying-sized glands lined by swollen cells with granular cytoplasm and hyperchromatic nuclei. HE × 250.

where there is foveolar hyperplasia and an infiltrate of plasma cells and lymphocytes.

The pathogenesis of this disorder is unclear. An allergic basis has been suggested because of the typical relapsing clinical course and high prevalence of eosinophilia in the blood. Lambert *et al.* (1978) were able to demonstrate increased numbers of IgE-containing plasma cells in the gastric mucosa adjacent to the erosions but this was not confirmed in another study (Tytgat *et al.*, 1982).

7.3 Eosinophilic gastritis

The stomach is the commonest site of involvement in eosinophilic gastroenteritis (also known as allergic gastroenteropathy). This uncommon condition results in a diffuse thickening of one or more segments of the gastrointestinal tract and predominantly affects young adults, approximately 25% of whom have a history of asthma or allergy (Johnstone and Morson, 1978). There is usually a peripheral blood eosinophilia and IgE levels may be elevated (Katz *et al.*, 1977; Caldwell *et al.*, 1979). Gastric disease results in symptoms of pyloric obstruction with vomiting or abdominal pain, and blood loss can lead to an iron-deficiency anaemia. Investigations may show malabsorption, protein loss, or both.

The principal changes on pathological examination of resected specimens have been a variable degree of oedema and infiltration by eosinophils, generally most marked in the submucosa but also affecting the muscle coats and subserosa. Gastroscopy has shown thickening and deformity of the antrum with narrowing of the pylorus and diminished peristalsis (Navab *et al.*, 1972), an appearance indistinguishable from infiltrating carcinoma. The mucosa may be reddened, swollen and contain erosions (Katz *et al.*, 1977). Biopsies show an intense infiltration of the lamina propria by eosinophils which can extend into the surface and glandular epithelium (Fig. 7.3). There is focal necrosis, and regenerative changes of the epithelium, resulting in nuclear enlargement, prominent nucleoli, decreased mucin content and increased numbers of mitoses, may be marked. Neutrophils can be conspicuous particularly in relation to areas of necrosis. There may be intestinal metaplasia. Gastric biopsy is of considerable value in diagnosis since the changes are diffuse, contrasting with the patchiness of small intestinal mucosal involvement (Leinbach and Rubin, 1970). The appearances however are not specific and marked eosinophilic infiltrates can occur in such conditions as Crohn's disease, tropical sprue (Floch *et al.*, 1963), chronic granulomatous disease of childhood (Griscom *et al.*, 1974), and accompanying peptic ulcers and carcinoma.

Occasional cases of localized disease, mostly in the small intestine,

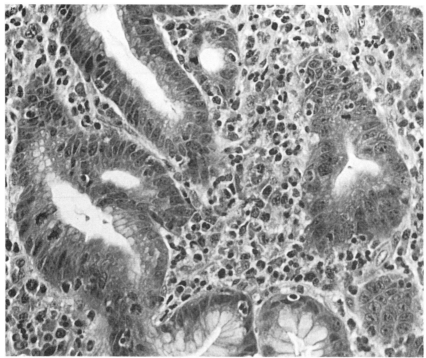

Fig. 7.3   Eosinophilic gastritis. Numerous eosinophils are present in the lamina propria and focally infiltrate the epithelium. HE × 375.

have been associated at the site of the lesion with the larvae of the anisakine nematode parasite of fish (Kuipers *et al.*, 1960; Watt *et al.*, 1979).

7.4   Fungal infection

Mycotic infection of the stomach is mostly due to *Candida albicans*, other strains of *Candida*, and *Torulopsis glabra* (Ahnlund *et al.*, 1967). Rare cases of phycomycosis (mucormycosis) have been reported (Deal and Johnson, 1969), and histoplasmosis may result in gastric ulceration as part of a systemic fatal disease (Pinkerton and Iverson, 1952; Nudelman and Rakatansky, 1966).

Gastric candidiasis has been diagnosed in approximately 1% of patients undergoing endoscopy (Minoli *et al.*, 1982). It mostly occurs as an opportunistic infection in debilitated individuals and is particularly associated with malignant neoplasms and the use of agents such as steroids, cytotoxic drugs and antibiotics. Occasional cases have been reported in uncompromised subjects (Nelson *et al.*, 1975). At endoscopy it may take the form of a white, yellow or greenish membrane of variable location and extension which can be easily removed to reveal an inflamed underlying mucosa, or consist of nodules a few millimetres in diameter mainly located in the antrum. The former type is often associated with oropharyngeal and/or oesophageal involvement. In addition, candidal infection of chronic peptic ulcers is common. In one series this was demonstrated in one-third of 72 consecutive surgically resected lesions. The presence of numerous fungi in clusters, sometimes with invasion of deep layers of the exudate, was identified in a poor-risk group with high post-operative mortality (Katzenstein and Maksem, 1979).

Brush cytology has a higher yield than biopsy in demonstrating fungal infection particularly in the membranous form. In biopsies, large numbers of organisms are easily detected in routinely stained sections (Fig. 7.4), but when scanty their demonstration is facilitated by a PAS or Grocott stain in suspected cases. Definitive identification of the organism involved is dependent on culture.

Occasionally a massive growth of fungi (phytobezoar) can occur in the

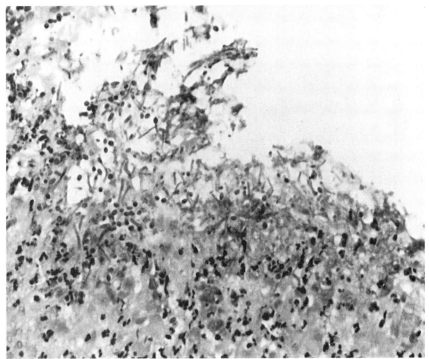

Fig. 7.4   Fungal hyphae and spores associated with slough from an ulcer. HE × 375.

stomach and be misinterpreted as necrotic tumour at endoscopy (Gabrielsson, 1971; Cipollini and Altilia, 1982). Most examples have been in individuals who have had a gastric resection in the past.

7.5　Granulomatous gastritis

Granulomas may be present in the gastric mucosa in sarcoidosis, a variety of infectious diseases, as a reaction to endogenous substances and to foreign material including indigestible food and sutures, and in Crohn's disease. Not uncommonly, however, no obvious predisposing factor is identified, so-called isolated granulomatous gastritis.

Symptomatic involvement of the intestinal tract in sarcoidosis is rare although granulomas were identified in 10% of gastric biopsies by Palmer (1958) in a study of patients with other evidence of sarcoid but without gastrointestinal symptoms. When symptoms have been present endoscopy has shown features varying from a distal gastritis with or without nodularity and mostly affecting the greater curve (Gould *et al.*, 1973; Jolobe and Montgomery, 1981) to ulceration and narrowing of the antrum (Sirak, 1954).

Tuberculosis, fungal diseases such as histoplasmosis and syphilis are all rare causes of granulomatous gastritis. Gastrointestinal involvement in tuberculosis most commonly implicates the ileo-caecal region and gastric disease is unusual even in those parts of the world where intestinal tuberculosis is prevalent (Misra *et al.*, 1982). Tuberculosis and cancer of the stomach may co-exist (Tanner and Swynnerton, 1955). Granulomas are necrotizing and often confluent but early forms may be indistinguishable from those in Crohn's disease or sarcoid. Stains for acid-fast bacilli are often negative and diagnosis may depend on culture or the presence of obvious disease elsewhere.

Disseminated histoplasmosis affecting the stomach can result in the development of giant gastric folds, with biopsies showing histoplasmaladen macrophages in the mucosa and submucosa (Fisher and Sanowski, 1978).

Rigid prominent gastric folds and multiple serpiginous erosions have been described in the secondary stage of gastric syphilis (Reisman *et al.*, 1975). Granulomas may be present but the most common finding is a dense infiltrate of plasma cells accompanied by numerous neutrophils, and spirochaetes may be demonstrated using immunofluorescence or in a Warthin-Starry preparation.

Foreign body granulomas can result from a reaction to exogenous substances such as suture material (Fig. 7.5) which penetrates the mucosa (Sanders and Woesner, 1972), and undigested food particles such as the integument of cereals which gain access to the stomach wall usually as a

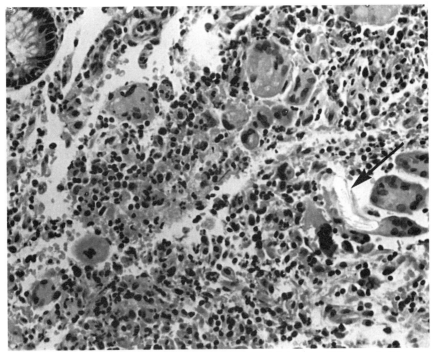

Fig. 7.5   Granulomatous reaction to suture material (arrowed) in gastric biopsy. HE × 150.

result of peptic ulceration. In these cases palisaded histiocytes and foreign body giant cells surround recognizable foreign material (Fig. 7.6). In some circumstances, however, a similar reaction occurs around unidentifiable amorphous granular material which may be eosinophilic or basophilic and can be calcified and resemble in shape an ova or worm. This probably represents a degenerative change of exposed smooth muscle or fibrous tissue in peptic ulcers produced by the digestive action of gastric juice (Sherman and Moran, 1954). A foreign body reaction to cholesterol emboli has been reported in biopsy material from an elderly patient with gastric telangiectases where it was postulated that the emboli may have induced the angiodysplastic lesions (Bank *et al.*, 1983). Mucin granulomas are another type of foreign body reaction to an endogenous substance and may occur in actively inflamed mucosa following glandular disruption. I have seen this change in resection specimens but not in biopsy material.

Symptomatic involvement of the stomach often accompanied by contiguous duodenal disease has been encountered in 1–2% of patients with Crohn's disease (Fielding *et al.*, 1970; Rutgeerts *et al.*, 1980). In nearly all reported cases ileal and/or colonic disease has also been present at the time of diagnosis of upper gastrointestinal disease. At endoscopy changes have predominated in the distal part of the stomach (Danzi *et al.*, 1976) and consist of enlarged rigid folds which may be nodular, the nodules often showing serpiginous erosion of their surface. A typical cobblestone pattern may be seen with fissuring ulceration surrounding nodules. Severe disease can give rise to such marked narrowing of the

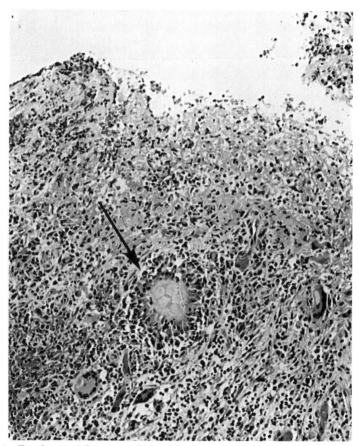

Fig. 7.6   Food material surrounded by histiocytes (arrowed). Ingested material is seen in adjacent foreign body giant cells. HE × 150.

Fig. 7.7   Crohn's disease. Inflamed antral mucosa with two epithelioid cell granulomas (arrowed). Patient had extensive ileal disease. HE × 90.

Fig. 7.8   Crohn's disease. There is considerable inflammation associated with intestinal metaplasia in this antral biopsy. Three small collections of macrophages (microgranulomas) are also present (arrowed). HE × 141.

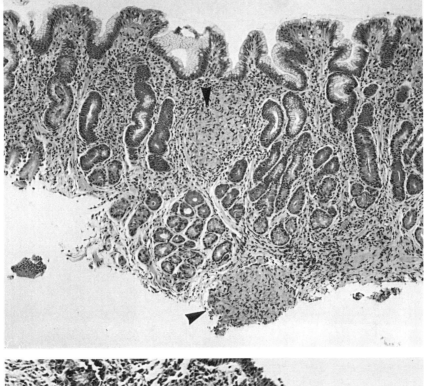

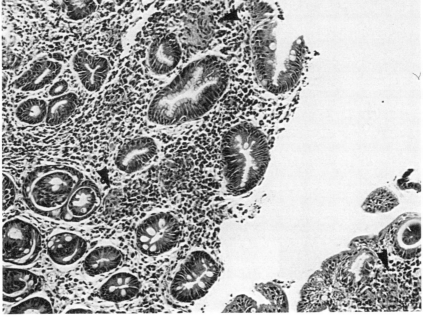

antrum and pre-pyloric region that the duodenum cannot be entered. In mild disease the appearances may suggest an unremarkable gastritis. Biopsies show non-specific inflammation which may however be very patchy, and this is best assessed when several samples are taken. The latter also increases the likelihood of detecting epithelioid cell granulomas (Figs 7.7 and 7.8), present in more than 50% of cases in one recent series (Rutgeerts *et al.*, 1980).

Isolated granulomatous gastritis (Fig. 7.9) refers to cases where non-

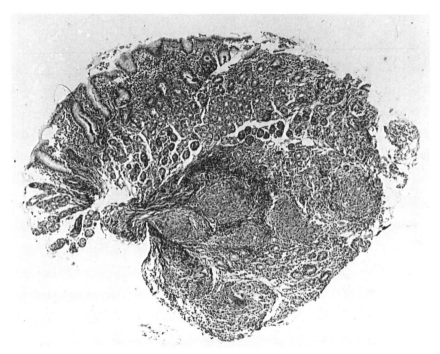

Fig. 7.9 Isolated granulomatous gastritis. Several granulomas in inflamed gastric body mucosa. Incidental finding in patient with dyspepsia. HE × 53.

caseating epithelioid cell granulomas have been present in the absence of recognized predisposing causes (Fahimi *et al.*, 1963). In a majority of reported cases there has been thickening and narrowing of the antrum and pre-pyloric region and patients have presented with obstructive symptoms. In some cases there has been an associated gastric ulcer or less commonly duodenal ulcer (Schinella and Ackert, 1979) but examination of resection specimens has shown that the granulomas are not intimately related to these. Peri-gastric lymph nodes have also contained granulomas.

References

Ahnlund, H. O., Pallin, B., Peterhoff, R. and Schönebeck, J. (1967), Mycosis of the stomach. *Acta Chir. Scand.*, **133**, 555–562.

Bank, S., Aftalion, B., Anfang, C. *et al.* (1983), Acquired angiodysplasia as a cause of gastric hemorrhage: a possible consequence of cholesterol embolization. *Am. J. Gastroenterol.*, **78**, 206–209.

Bron, B. A., Deyhle, P., Pelloni, S. *et al.* (1977), Phlegmonous gastritis diagnosed by endoscopic snare biopsy. *Dig. Dis.*, **22**, 729–733.

Caldwell, J. H., Sharma, H. M., Hurtubise, P. E. and Colwell, D. L. (1979), Eosinophilic gastroenteritis in extreme allergy. Immunopathological comparison with nonallergic gastrointestinal disease. *Gastroenterology*, **77**, 560–564.

Cipollini, F. and Altilia, F. (1982), Mycetoma of the gastric stump *Gastrointest. Endosc.*, **28**, 220–221. (letter).

Danzi, J. T., Farmer, R. G., Sullivan, B. H. Jr. and Rankin, G. B. (1976), Endoscopic features of gastroduodenal Crohn's disease. *Gastroenterology*, **70**, 9–13.

Deal, W. B. and Johnson, J. E. III (1969), Gastric phycomycosis. Report of a case and review of the literature. *Gastroenterology*, **57**, 579–586.

Fahimi, H. D., Deren, J. J., Gottlieb, L. S. and Zamcheck, N. (1963), Isolated granulomatous gastritis: its relationship to disseminated sarcoidosis and regional enteritis. *Gastroenterology*, **45**, 161–175.

Fielding, J. F., Toye, D. K. M., Beton, D. C. and Cooke, W. T. (1970), Crohn's disease of the stomach and duodenum. *Gut*, **11**, 1001–1006.

Fisher, J. R. and Sanowski, R. A. (1978), Disseminated histoplasmosis producing hypertrophic gastric folds. *Dig. Dis.*, **23**, 282–285.

Floch, M. H., Thomassen, R. W., Cox, R. S. Jr. and Sheehy, T. W. (1963), The gastric mucosa in tropical sprue. *Gastroenterology*, **44**, 567–577.

Gabrielsson, N. (1971), Growth of yeast-like fungi in the stomach. A gastrophotographic and roentgenographic study. *Endoscopy*, **2**, 66–73.

Gould, S. R., Handley, A. J. and Barnardo, D. E. (1973), Rectal and gastric involvement in a case of sarcoidosis. *Gut*, **14**, 971–973.

Griscom, N. T., Kirkpatrick, J. A. Jr., Girdany, B. R. *et al.* (1974), Gastric antral narrowing in chronic granulomatous disease of childhood. *Pediatrics*, **54**, 456–460.

Isaacson, P. (1982), Biopsy appearances easily mistaken for malignancy in gastrointestinal endoscopy. *Histopathology*, **6**, 377–389.

Johnstone, J. M. and Morson, B. C. (1978), Eosinophilic gastroenteritis. *Histopathology*, **2**, 335–348.

Jolobe, O. M. P. and Montgomery, R. D. (1981), Gastric sarcoidosis *Gastrointest. Endosc.*, **27**, 199–200. (letter).

Katz, A. J., Goldman, H. and Grand, R. J. (1977), Gastric mucosal biopsy in eosinophilic (allergic) gastroenteritis. *Gastroenterology*, **73**, 705–709.

Katzenstein, A-L. A. and Maksem, J. (1979), Candidal infection of gastric ulcers. Histology, incidence, and clinical significance. *Am. J. Clin. Pathol.*, **71**, 137–141.

Kuipers, F. C., van Thiel, P. H., Rodenburg, W. *et al.* (1960), Eosinophilic phlegmon of the alimentary canal caused by a worm. *Lancet*, **ii**, 1171–1173.

Lambert, R., Andre, C., Moulinier, B. and Bugnon, B. (1978), Diffuse varioliform gastritis. *Digestion*, **17**, 159–167.

Leinbach, G. E. and Rubin, C. E. (1970), Eosinophilic gastroenteritis: a simple reaction to food allergens? *Gastroenterology*, **59**, 874–889.

Miller, A. I., Smith, B. and Rogers, A. I. (1975), Phlegmonous gastritis. *Gastroenterology*, **68**, 231–238.

Minoli, G., Terruzzi, V., Butti, G. *et al.* (1982), Gastric candidiasis: an endoscopic and histological study in 26 patients. *Gastrointest. Endosc.*, **28**, 59–61.

Misra, R. C., Agarwal, S. K., Prakash, P. *et al.* (1982), Gastric tuberculosis. *Endoscopy*, **14**, 235–237.

Morgan, A. G., McAdam, W. A. F., Pyrah, R. D. and Tinsley, E. G. F. (1976), Multiple recurring gastric erosions (aphthous ulcers). *Gut*, **17**, 633–639.

Navab, F., Kleinman, M. S., Algazy, K. *et al.* (1972), Endoscopic diagnosis of eosinophilic gastritis. *Gastrointest. Endosc.*, **19**, 67–69.

Nelson, R. S., Bruni, H. C. and Goldstein, H. M. (1975), Primary gastric candidiasis in uncompromised subjects. *Gastrointest. Endosc.*, **22**, 92–94.

Nudelman, H. L. and Rakatansky, H. (1966), Gastric histoplasmosis. A case report. *J. Am. Med. Assoc.*, **195**, 134–136.

Palmer, E. D. (1958), Note on silent sarcoidosis of the gastric mucosa. *J. Lab. Clin. Med.*, **52**, 231–234.

Pinkerton, H. and Iverson, S. (1952), Histoplasmosis: three fatal cases with disseminated sarcoid-like lesions. *Arch. Intern. Med.*, **90**, 456–467.

Reisman, T. N., Leverett, F. L., Hudson, J. R. and Kaiser, M. H. (1975), Syphilitic gastropathy. *Dig. Dis.*, **20**, 588–593.

Roesch, W. (1978), Erosions of the upper gastrointestinal tract. *Clin. Gastroenterol.*, **7**, 623–634.

Rutgeerts, P., Onette, E., Vantrappen, G. *et al.* (1980), Crohn's disease of the stomach and duodenum: a clinical study with emphasis on the value of endoscopy and endoscopic biopsies. *Endoscopy*, **12**, 288–294.

Sanders, I. and Woesner, M. E. (1972), 'Stitch' granuloma: a consideration in the differential diagnosis of the intramural gastric tumor. *Am. J. Gastroenterol.*, **57**, 558–562.

Schinella, R. A. and Ackert, J. (1979), Isolated granulomatous disease of the stomach. Report of three cases presenting as incidental findings in gastrectomy specimens. *Am. J. Gastroenterol.*, **72**, 30–35.

Sherman, F. E. and Moran, T. J. (1954), Granulomas of stomach. I. Response to injury of muscle and fibrous tissue of wall of human stomach. *Am. J. Clin. Pathol.*, **24**, 415–421.

Sirak, H. D. (1954), Boeck's sarcoid of the stomach simulating linitis plastica. Report of a case and comparison with twelve recorded cases. *Arch. Surg.*, **69**, 769–776.

Tanner, N. C. and Swynnerton, B. F. (1955), Gastric tuberculosis associated with gastric carcinoma. *Br. J. Surg.*, **43**, 573–576.

Tytgat, G. N., Dekker, W. and Balk, T. (1982), Immunologic and ultrastructural investigations in chronic erosive varioliform gastritis. *Gastroenterology*, **82**, 1200 (abstract).

Watt, I. A., McLean, N. R., Girdwood, R. W. A. *et al.* (1979), Eosinophilic gastroenteritis associated with a larval anisakine nematode. *Lancet*, **ii**, 893–894.

8 Gastric polyps and thickened folds

8.1 Gastric polyps

The clinical term polyp is used to describe any focal lesion which projects above the surface of the surrounding mucosa, and used alone gives no indication of its nature. Gastric polyps are found in only about 0.4% of autopsies (Plachta and Speer, 1957) but are present in up to 5% of routine endoscopies although many of them are very small (Rösch, 1980). Although a polypoid appearance can result from unaffected islands of mucosa occurring in a diffusely atrophic stomach (these are more properly termed pseudo-polyps), in common usage the term implies a substantive process occurring in the mucosa or less commonly submucosa. Most consideration will be given here to mucosal polyps since they are far commoner and the usual source of material for the pathologist. This may be either as biopsy samples, or, if the whole lesion is removed, as a polypectomy specimen. Although examination of the entire lesion is preferable and biopsy samples may not be representative, gastric polypectomy is a relatively new technique and presents more difficulties for the endoscopist than the same procedure in the large bowel, since the polyps are frequently sessile and often quite vascular.

The classification of gastric mucosal polyps is a matter of debate, but from a clinical point of view, the most important distinction is between the neoplastic and non-neoplastic groups. Here they will be considered under four headings – hyperplastic, neoplastic, hamartomatous, and a miscellaneous group.

8.1.1 Hyperplastic polyps

These are the commonest type of gastric polyp, constituting from 50 to 90% of the total (Ming and Goldman, 1965; Tomasulo, 1971). They are smooth surfaced or only slightly lobulated, oval or hemispherical in shape, and rarely greater than 1.5 cm in diameter. Their surface is often eroded. The majority are sessile but larger polyps may be pedunculated. They can be single or multiple and may occur anywhere in the stomach although commonest in the antrum. When multiple they may be widely scattered, or confined to one area, sometimes being concentrated at the junction of the body and antral mucosa.

Histologically they consist of markedly hyperplastic and elongated foveolae in which intraluminal infolding and branching is frequent and cystic dilatation almost invariable in the deeper parts of the polyp (Figs 8.1 and 8.2). The lining cells consist of a single layer of regularly arranged hypertrophied foveolar epithelium containing abundant neutral mucin. In some areas the cells may be cuboidal with granular eosinophilic cytoplasm (Muto and Oota, 1970). Small groups of pyloric type glands are present beneath the proliferating foveolae and connect with some of them. Parietal and chief cells are uncommon even when the polyp occurs in body mucosa. Intestinal metaplasia can occur but is rarely a conspicuous feature and when present usually focal (Figs 8.3 and 8.4). Bundles of smooth muscle fibres growing into the polyp from the muscularis mucosae are frequently seen and the lamina propria is variably oedematous and infiltrated by plasma cells and lymphocytes. Lymphoid aggregates with germinal centres can sometimes be present. At sites of erosion there is a fibrinopurulent exudate associated with the

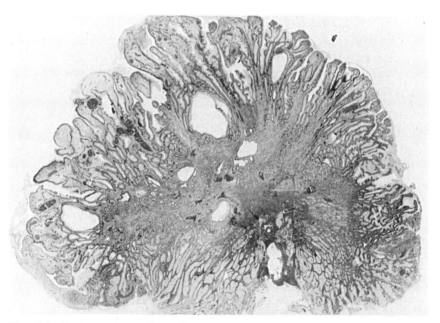

Fig. 8.1 Regenerative polyp. Foveolar hyperplasia and cyst formation are conspicuous. HE × 10.

presence of numerous acute inflammatory cells and proliferated capillaries in the subjacent tissues. In such areas bizarre-appearing, pleomorphic cells with hyperchromatic nuclei and prominent nucleoli may be seen scattered or in small groups in the stroma (Fig. 8.5). Some of them show mitoses. These are regenerative and not malignant cells, although the cell type from which they are derived is uncertain (Dirschmid *et al.*, 1984). The mucosa adjacent to a hyperplastic polyp usually shows similar though less marked changes of hypertrophy and hyperplasia of the foveolar cells, and mild to moderate inflammation with or without focal intestinal metaplasia and cyst formation, so that there is no clear demarcation between the two.

Because of their histological features and the fact that they can develop

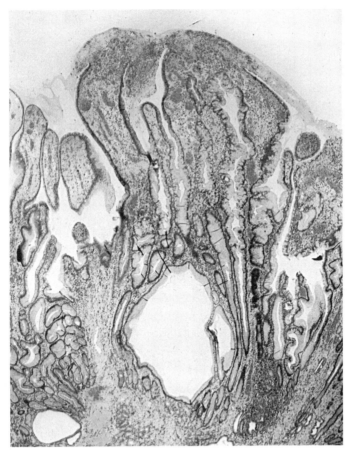

Fig. 8.2 Focal erosion of surface. Elongated and often tortuous foveolae and moderate inflammation in the stroma of the polyp. HE × 27.

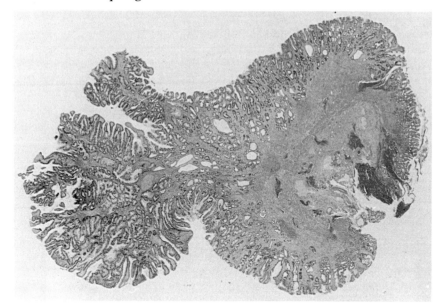

Fig. 8.3   Regenerative polyp. Low power view of antral polyp. HE × 7.

at the site of, or bordering, ulcers and erosions (Mori *et al.*, 1971) and at gastroenterostomy stomas (Section 6.4) it seems that these polyps arise on the basis of excessive regeneration following mucosal damage. Hence their alternative name of regenerative polyps.

A distinctive feature of a minority of hyperplastic polyps has been a concentric infolding of the papillary surface epithelium which macroscopically corresponds to a central dimple. These polyps, which have been separately categorized by Nakamura (1970), are usually multiple and arranged in a band in the fundic mucosa adjacent to the pyloric antrum. They probably result from over-exuberant healing of gastric erosions. Another classification separates those polyps with foveolar hyperplasia only and which tend to be small, from larger polyps in which there is in addition stromal and glandular hyperplasia and referred to as hyperplasiogenous polyps (Elster, 1974). The essential change however in all of them appears similar, varying only in degree.

Although there is general agreement that the malignant potential of hyperplastic polyps is low, occasional examples of malignant change have been reported (Nakamura, 1970; Kozuka *et al.*, 1977; Remmele and Kolb, 1978). On the other hand these polyps are often associated with an independent carcinoma elsewhere in the stomach, being found in 10% of cases of advanced gastric cancer and in 18% of cases of early gastric carcinoma in one report (Rösch, 1980).

8.1.2 Neoplastic polyps

These are uncommon and consist of adenomas and polypoid carcinomas (types I, IIa and IIa + IIc early gastric cancers – Section 9.2.1). Occasionally carcinoid tumours arise in the stomach and often take the form of a polyp.

(a) *Adenomas.* These are soft velvety lesions which are sessile or broad based. They are mostly single and predominate in the antrum. In surgical series they have often been large with an average diameter of 4 cm (Ming and Goldman, 1965) and sometimes reach enormous proportions. They have an irregular surface with papillary projections separated by deep

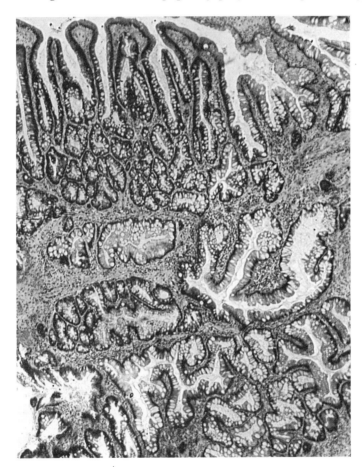

Fig. 8.4 Detail of Fig. 8.3 shows large numbers of goblet cells. Intestinal metaplasia is not usually a conspicuous feature of such polyps. HE × 37.5.

fissures. Direct observation of the stomach at endoscopy however has resulted in the recognition of smaller, flatter, usually lobulated adenomas often with a slightly depressed centre which protrude into the lumen by only a few millimetres and which have been referred to rather confusingly as borderline lesions or as lesions with atypical epithelium (Sugano *et al.*, 1971). Unlike hyperplastic polyps, adenomas have a significant potential for malignant change which in reported series has averaged 40% (Ming, 1977).

Larger adenomas have a villous or tubulo-villous architecture (Fig. 8.6) but the small flat lesions have a tubular pattern (Fig. 8.7). Their epithelium consists of crowded, columnar cells with large hyperchromatic elongated nuclei and amphophilic to slightly basophilic cytoplasm in

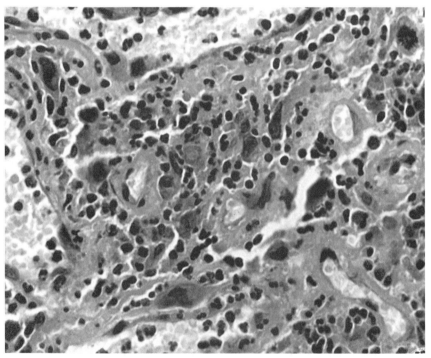

Fig. 8.5 Regenerative polyp. Large pleomorphic cells with hyperchromatic nuclei. Mitosis at top right. HE × 600.

Fig. 8.6 Adenoma. Tubulo-villous configuration. Cystic change is prominent. This 2 cm diameter lesion was present in the fundus. HE × 5.
Fig. 8.7 Adenoma. Small sessile antral polyp composed of moderately dysplastic epithelium with a tubular pattern. Note obvious transition between dysplastic and non-dysplastic epithelium. HE × 60.

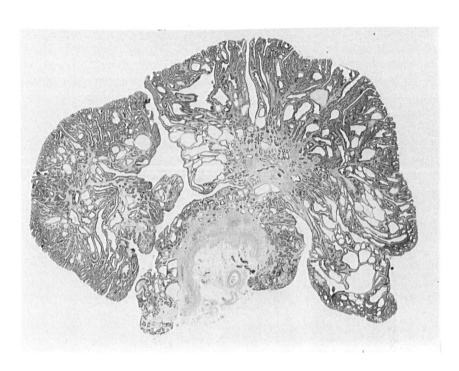

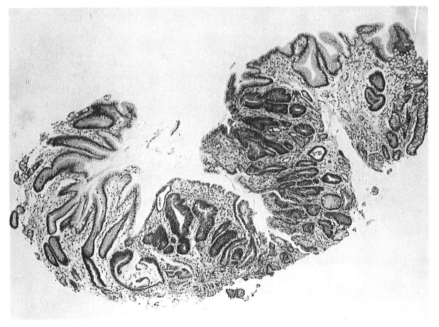

which mucus is either absent or scant. Pseudostratification of nuclei and frequent mitoses are seen. Occasional goblet cells can be present along with Paneth and argentaffin cells. Within the polyp small islands of uninvolved but usually metaplastic epithelium occur and occasional pyloric glands are present at the base. In the sessile tubular adenomas (borderline lesion) cystic dilatation of glands is frequent deep to the dysplastic epithelium. There is a sharp cut-off between adenomatous epithelium and that of the adjacent mucosa which often shows atrophic gastritis with intestinal metaplasia. This and the features of the adenomas themselves suggest that they have originated from metaplastic glands (Morson, 1955).

Based on the degree of cytological atypia and on the disorganization of the mucosal architecture, adenomas may be subjectively categorized as showing mild (Fig. 8.8), moderate or severe (Fig. 8.9) epithelial dysplasia.

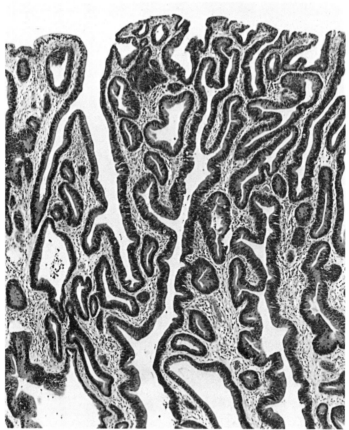

Fig. 8.8   Adenoma. Detail of Fig. 8.6 shows minor epithelial dysplasia. HE × 60.

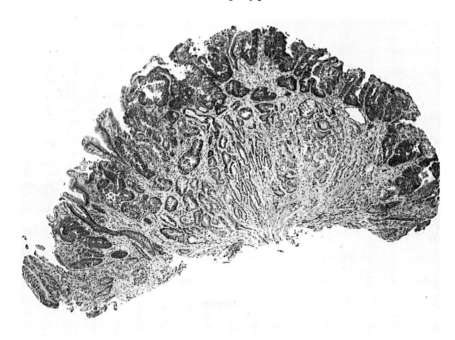

Fig. 8.9   Adenoma. Severely dysplastic epithelium is confined to the superficial part of the mucosa. HE × 51.

Examination of multiple sections is essential, particularly when more marked degrees of dysplasia are present, to detect any areas of invasion of neoplastic cells through the basal membrane of the glands and pits. The distinction between highly differentiated intramucosal adenocarcinoma and severe dysplasia in an adenoma on histological grounds (Fig. 8.10) is often particularly difficult (Section 9.1).

An endoscopic and histological follow-up study of 85 adenomas, most of which were under 2 cm in size, for periods up to 12 years showed that malignant change occurred in 9 (11%). Seven of these were over 2 cm in diameter and three of them had shown an increase in size during the period of follow-up. Co-existent gastric cancers, five of which were early gastric cancers (egc) of the protruded type, were present in 14 of the 74 patients studied (Kamiya *et al.*, 1982). In another study of elevated types of egc (Johansen, 1979), which are usually well-differentiated tumours, features suggestive of an origin in an adenoma were seen in a majority.

Since individual adenomas may show varying degrees of epithelial dysplasia it should always be borne in mind that endoscopic biopsies may not sample areas with the most marked changes which may occur focally within the tumour. In general it can be said that because of their malignant potential these uncommon lesions should be removed, by total or piecemeal endoscopic polypectomy, if feasible, or by surgical resection. This particularly applies to larger tumours and those with a severe degree of epithelial dysplasia. However, since adenomas tend to occur in older age groups, regular endoscopic follow-up with multiple biopsies may be more appropriate in the individual case.

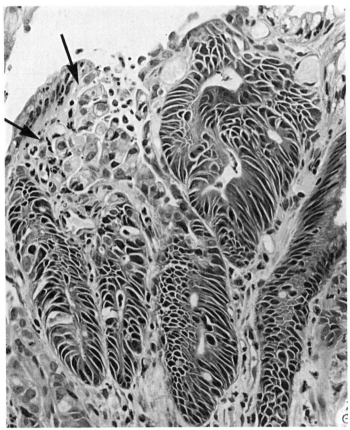

Fig. 8.10 Adenoma. Detail of Fig. 8.9 shows severe dysplasia with apparent spillage of neoplastic cells into the lamina propria (arrowed). This probably represents a focus of intramucosal carcinoma. HE × 330.

(b) *Carcinoid tumours*. The term carcinoid is given to tumours with a distinct morphology and derived from one or more of a heterogeneous population of endocrine cells. Alternative names have been APUD-omas (see Andrew, 1982) or more simply endocrine cell tumours. A more specific classification is based on their cell of origin or hormone product e.g. gastrin cell tumour or gastrinoma.

Approximately 5% of gastrointestinal tract carcinoids occur in the stomach (Hajdu *et al.*, 1974) and in this site they are commonly polypoid. The majority arise in the antrum. They may be covered by intact mucosa or show central ulceration, and larger tumours may be grossly indistinguishable from ulcerated adenocarcinoma. Multiple tumours occur in 6–7% of cases. Because they arise deep in the mucosa, superficial endoscopic biopsies may not obtain diagnostic material and polypectomy or button-hole biopsy is likely to be more successful (Seifert and Elster, 1977).

Histologically they are composed of small uniform cells which are arranged in nests and infiltrating strands, or have an anastomosing ribbon-like pattern (Figs 8.11 and 8.12). Occasionally a tubular or acinar arrangement is seen. There is a loose, vascular, connective tissue stroma, which rarely may be hyalinized, and tumour cells may be aggregated around sinusoids to form rosettes. There is often associated hyperplasia of the gastric glands and pits. The majority of gastric carcinoids are argyrophilic with the Grimelius technique, although this may only be

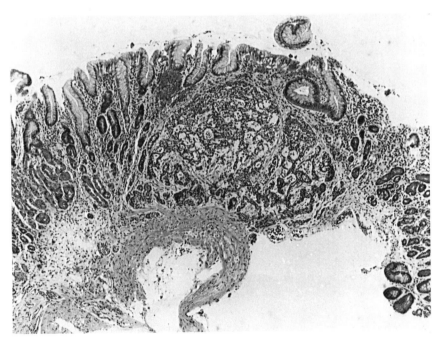

Fig. 8.11 Carcinoid tumour. A circumscribed nest of tumour cells was an incidental finding in a random antral biopsy. HE × 60.

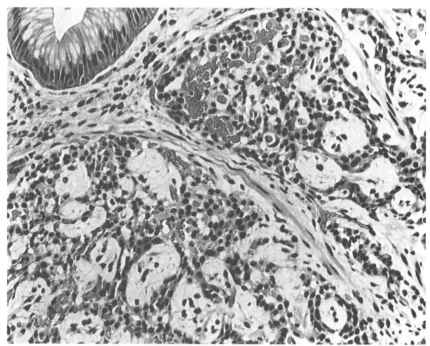

Fig. 8.12   Carcinoid tumour. Detail of Fig. 8.11 shows small uniform cells with a pseudo-acinar pattern. HE × 277.

demonstrable when fixatives such as Bouin's solution have been used. They are rarely argentaffin positive (Jones and Dawson, 1977; Wilander *et al.*, 1977). Alpha-l-antitrypsin has been demonstrated in some of these tumours (Ray *et al.*, 1982).

Several reports have documented the presence of one or more carcinoid tumours and/or diffuse hyperplasia of endocrine cells in the body of the stomach in patients with pernicious anaemia (Pestana *et al.*, 1963; Larsson *et al.*, 1978; Goldman *et al.*, 1981; Hodges *et al.*, 1981; Section 6.3), atrophic gastritis (Rubin, 1973; Gueller and Haddad, 1975; Russo *et al.*, 1980), following gastrojejunostomy (Lemmer, 1942; Bordi *et al.*, 1976) and in the Zollinger-Ellison syndrome (Solcia *et al.*, 1970; Bordi *et al.*, 1974). In all these conditions there is a raised serum gastrin and it is presumed that this is the stimulus for endocrine cell proliferation. On the basis of their staining properties and ultrastructural characteristics they have been characterized as enterochromaffin-like (ECL) cells (Bordi *et al.*, 1976; Hodges *et al.*, 1981), although in one recent report multiple tumours in the fundus of a man with pernicious anaemia contained gastrin (Morgan *et al.*, 1983), and tumours composed of a mixed population of endocrine cells (ECL cells and various subtypes of enterochromaffin cells) have also been reported (Larsson *et al.*, 1978).

Gastric carcinoid tumours have only rarely been associated with systemic effects of the carcinoid syndrome (Christodoulopoulos and Klotz, 1961). They may elaborate 5-hydroxytryptophan and histamine, but only rarely serotonin (Chejfec and Gould, 1977; Wilander *et al.*, 1979). Very occasionally tumours have produced ACTH and resulted in Cushing's syndrome (Hirata *et al.*, 1976; Marcus *et al.*, 1980).

In general these tumours are slow growing and, even when metastases to regional lymph nodes have occurred, may be compatible with long-term survival (Lattes and Grossi, 1956). Recent studies have demonstrated that not all endocrine cell tumours in the stomach exhibit typical features and that a significant proportion of resected tumours, initially considered to be adenocarcinomas, represent atypical or poorly differentiated carcinoid tumours (Rogers and Murphy, 1979; Sweeney and McDonnell, 1980). Histologically they may take the form of sheets of cells without a recognizable pattern or even consist in part of spindle cells with a very vascular stroma resembling a sarcoma. It is important to make the diagnosis in these cases since, because of their relatively indolent course, an aggressive surgical policy even in the case of advanced tumours is likely to contribute to prolonged survival. Repeat endoscopy and biopsy may be indicated in these circumstances when samples can be placed in fixatives best suited for ultrastructural examination and for the demonstration of endocrine cell properties.

8.1.3   Hamartomatous polyps

(a) *Peutz-Jeghers polyps.* Endoscopy has shown that polyps with a characteristic histological appearance are present in the stomach in nearly half of those individuals with the Peutz-Jeghers syndrome (Utsunomiya *et al.*, 1975). In this site they are lobulated, rarely pedunculated, and mostly number less than ten. Although usually found incidentally, gastric polyps may bleed and there is a low but definite risk of malignant change (Dodds *et al.*, 1972; Cochet *et al.*, 1979), so that regular endoscopy with removal of any polyps present has been recommended in the management of patients with this uncommon disorder (Williams *et al.*, 1982). Histologically, the characteristic feature is the tree-like branching of the muscularis mucosae with overlying mucosa being of normal or hyperplastic antral or fundal type depending on the site of the polyp (Fig. 8.13). As well as the typical polyp, hyperplastic polyps may also occur in this condition (Fig. 8.14).

(b) *Juvenile polyps.* As the name suggests, juvenile polyps occur predominantly in children and adolescents and when solitary or few in number mostly affect the large bowel, particularly the lower rectum. When numerous, the upper gastrointestinal tract is frequently involved. Familial and non-familial cases of juvenile polyposis have been described, and in one recent report of the former type, multiple polyps were restricted to the stomach (Watanabe *et al.*, 1979). Multiple gastric polyps have resulted in chronic and severe loss of blood and protein (Ruymann, 1969; Watanabe *et al.*, 1979).

Characteristically, the polyps are round, smooth surfaced and may show evidence of haemorrhage. In the stomach they have been more numerous in the antrum or restricted to that site (Goodman *et al.*, 1979) and larger lesions have been pedunculated. Microscopical examination

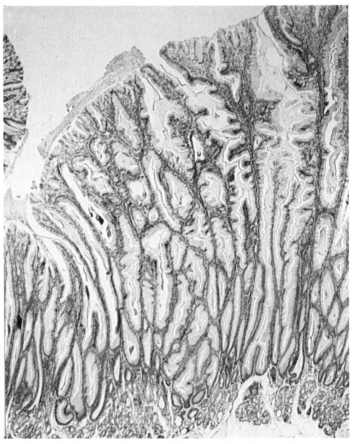

Fig. 8.13 Peutz-Jeghers syndrome. Thin strands of smooth muscle extend between enormously lengthened foveolae. HE × 30.

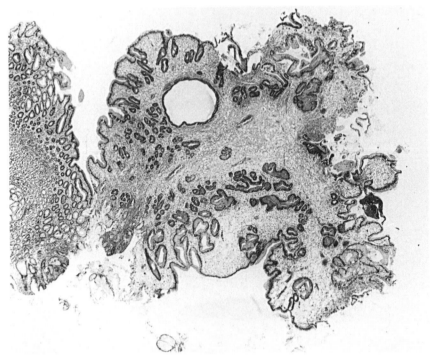

Fig. 8.14 Elongated and branched foveolae and cyst formation with an oedematous stroma. Antral polyp in patient with Peutz-Jeghers syndrome. HE × 16.

shows cystically dilated glands lined by foveolar epithelium lying in an abundant oedematous lamina propria infiltrated by variable numbers of inflammatory cells (Fig. 8.15). The smooth surface of the polyp may be focally eroded. Rarely foci of cartilaginous or osseous metaplasia are present in the stroma. Fibres of the muscularis mucosae are absent from the polyp. In some cases of juvenile polyposis, the gastric lesions have been indistinguishable histologically from hyperplastic polyps (Goodman *et al.*, 1979).

The malignant potential of juvenile polyps is low although there are reports describing areas of epithelial dysplasia and even of invasive carcinoma in otherwise typical polyps of the large bowel in cases of juvenile polyposis (Stemper *et al.*, 1975; Beacham *et al.*, 1978; Goodman *et al.*, 1979; Grigioni *et al.*, 1981; Järvinen and Franssila, 1984). However this sequence has not so far been documented in the stomach.

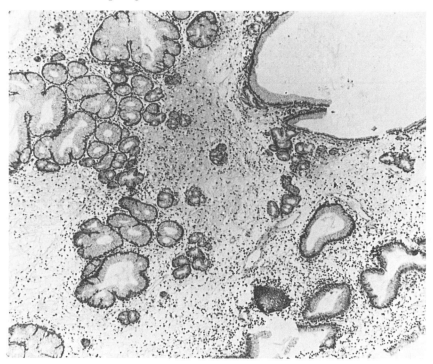

Fig. 8.15   Juvenile polyp. HE × 60.

8.1.4   *Miscellaneous mucosal polyps*

(a) *Cronkhite-Canada syndrome*. In this rare disorder of unknown aetiology and without any familial tendency there is generalized gastrointestinal polyposis associated with skin pigmentation, alopecia and atrophy of the nails (Cronkhite and Canada, 1955). There have been approximately 80 cases reported in the literature (Ikeda *et al.*, 1981). The major symptom is watery diarrhoea which can precede (Johnston *et al.*, 1962; Jarnum and Jensen, 1966) or follow the ectodermal changes (Ali *et al.*, 1980) and which can give rise to marked electrolyte disturbances and hypoproteinaemia. The majority of patients have been middle-aged or elderly and there is a slight male predominance.

Endoscopically the polyps have a glistening, glassy appearance due to the presence of mucous cysts and may be sessile or finger-like in appearance or result in irregular, polypoid, nodular folds resembling the appearances seen for example, with a diffusely infiltrating malignant lymphoma. Histologically there is intense oedema of the lamina propria usually associated with an increased cellularity, and elongation and tortuosity of the foveolae with marked cystic change in the pits and glands (Figs 8.16 and 8.17). Cysts may rupture and result in inflammation and the presence of muciphages in the lamina propria (Fig. 8.18). The histological appearances are not specific and may be indistinguishable from those of juvenile polyps (Kindbloom *et al.*, 1977).

(b) *Fundic glandular cysts*. This recently described polyp (Elster, 1976) has been observed in up to 1.5% of routine gastroscopies when carefully looked for (Sipponen *et al.*, 1983). The majority of cases have been in middle-aged women and no specific association with other gastric diseases has been noted. Together with adenomas and hyperplastic polyps (Utsunomiya *et al.*, 1974; Ranzi *et al.*, 1981) this lesion has also been reported in the stomachs of patients with familial adenomatosis coli (Watanabe *et al.*, 1978; Eichenberger *et al.*, 1980; Burt *et al.*, 1984).

Occasionally single, but often numbering in the order of 15 to 30, they appear endoscopically as clusters of small, mostly sessile lesions (up to about 5 mm in diameter) with a glassy transparent appearance, and are restricted to the body and fundus of the stomach, i.e. within the acid-secreting area (Tatsuta *et al.*, 1981). One case has also been described in heterotopic gastric body mucosa in the duodenal bulb (Elster *et al.*, 1977). Histologically, cysts of variable size are present at different levels of the

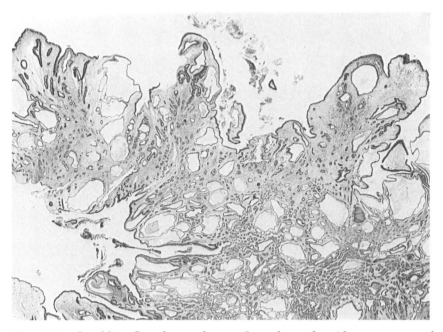

Fig. 8.16 Cronkhite-Canada syndrome. Irregular polypoid appearance of mucosa. HE × 6.

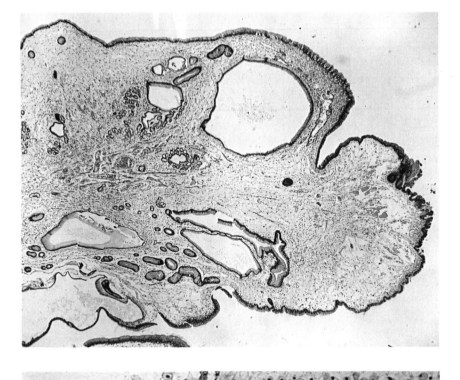

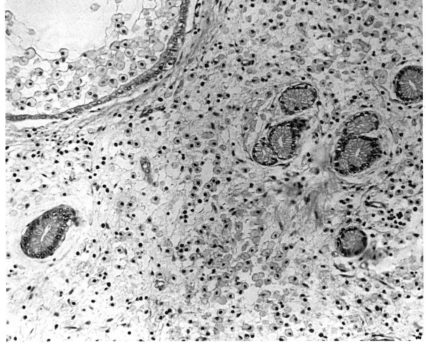

gastric glands admixed with normal glands (Figs 8.19 and 8.20). These cysts are often interconnected and are lined by mucin-secreting cells, rather atrophic parietal cells and some chief cells, although the latter are not conspicuous. There is usually no associated inflammation.

The histogenesis of this type of polyp is unclear but the appearances suggest that it is a hamartoma. Follow-up has shown that the number and size of polyps tends to remain unchanged, but in some cases spontaneous disappearance over a period of several months or a few years has been observed (Iida *et al.*, 1980).

8.1.5   Non-epithelial polyps

Various mesenchymal tumours may take the form of a hemispherical or occasionally a pedunculated gastric polyp covered by smooth stretched

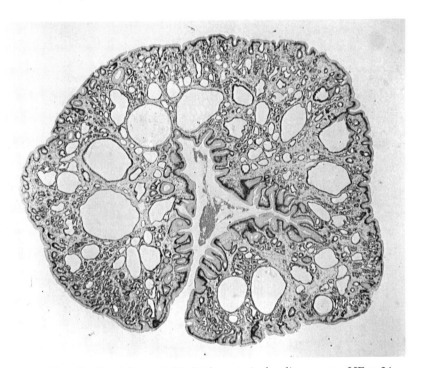

Fig. 8.19   Fundic glandular cyst. Multiple cysts in fundic mucosa. HE × 24.

Fig. 8.17   Cronkhite-Canada syndrome. Detail of Fig. 8.16 showing foveolar lengthening and cyst formation with an oedematous stroma. HE × 22.
Fig. 8.18   Cronkhite-Canada syndrome. Numerous muciphages in the lumen of a cystic gland and in the stroma. HE × 150.

mucosa in which central ulceration is frequent. The commonest types are smooth muscle tumours (Section 9.5) followed by neurogenic tumours. Metastatic tumours, which are frequently multiple, may give a similar endoscopic appearance (Dutta and Costa, 1979). Non-neoplastic polyps include aberrant or ectopic pancreatic tissue (Section 12.1.3), which in the stomach occurs mostly on the greater curve in the antrum, and inflammatory fibroid polyps. The stomach is the commonest site in the gastrointestinal tract for this uncommon lesion, which has also been called eosinophil granuloma, gastric fibroma with eosinophil infiltration, gastric submucosal granuloma, polypoid eosinophilic gastritis and inflammatory pseudotumour. In the majority of cases a single, smooth-surfaced

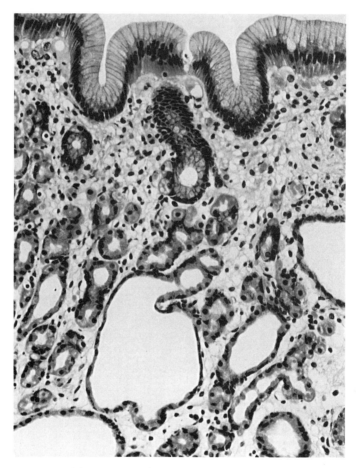

Fig. 8.20 Cysts of fundic glands lined by flattened epithelium which includes parietal cells. HE × 217.

oval polyp with a short pedicle which often shows surface erosion has been present in the pyloric antrum. Abdominal pain has been the commonest symptom. Histologically, inflammatory fibroid polyps consist of non-encapsulated, extremely vascular and usually loose connective tissue in the submucosa infiltrated by variable numbers of eosinophils, plasma cells, basophils, lymphocytes and histiocytes (Fig. 8.21). The latter two cell types may form aggregates, but true granuloma formulation is rare. Blood vessels range from capillaries to larger thin or thick-walled channels which are often surrounded by a zone of loose connective tissue giving a characteristic whorled pattern. These lesions have been mis-diagnosed as haemangiopericytomas (Helwig and Ranier, 1952).

The precise nature and aetiology of this polyp is unknown. Occasional cases have arisen at the edge of a peptic ulcer (Vanek, 1949) or carcinoma, and a jejunal polyp has been described following mucosal damage after a saline emetic (Calam *et al.*, 1982) suggesting an over-reactive healing process. A proposed neurogenic origin (Goldman and Friedman, 1967)

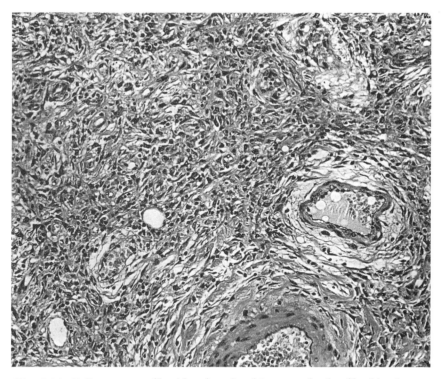

Fig. 8.21 Inflammatory fibroid polyp. In this example the fibroblastic component is denser than normal. Note large numbers of blood vessels. HE × 150.

appears unlikely and is not substantiated by ultrastructural examination (Williams, 1981). The suggestion that inflammatory fibroid polyps may be a localized variant of eosinophilic gastroenteritis (Ureles *et al.*, 1961) has been convincingly refuted (Johnstone and Morson, 1978).

8.2   Thickened gastric folds

Enlarged or thickened gastric folds on radiological examination or at endoscopy occur in a variety of disorders and may be associated with a nodular or polypoid appearance of the mucosa. État mammelonné is an uncommon variation of the normal where the gastric rugae are thickened and have a fine cobblestone appearance. Pathological conditions resulting in thickened gastric folds include infections due to tuberculosis, syphilis (Section 7.5) and fungi such as Candida and Histoplasma (Section 7.4), Crohn's disease (Section 7.5), eosinophilic gastroenteritis (Section 7.3), lymphangiectasia, and malignant infiltrations by carcinoma or lymphoma. Gastric varices also result in this appearance and need to be borne in mind by the endoscopist before he reaches for the biopsy forceps! Two other conditions which give rise to giant folds which are characteristically restricted to the body mucosa are the Zollinger-Ellison syndrome and Menetrier's disease.

8.2.1   *Zollinger-Ellison syndrome*

As originally described this comprised intractable peptic ulcer disease, acid hypersecretion and islet cell tumours of the pancreas (Zollinger and Ellison, 1955). The gastric secretagogue present in these tumours was later identified as gastrin (Gregory *et al.*, 1967). Although gastrinomas predominantly occur in the pancreas, either as single or multiple lesions, in approximately 10% of cases they arise in the duodenum, most commonly the second part (Oberhelman, 1972), and rarely the stomach (Royston *et al.*, 1972; Larsson *et al.*, 1973). Hyperplasia of antral gastrin (G) cells (also termed pseudo Zollinger-Ellison syndrome) results in an identical clinical picture (Polak *et al.*, 1972; Friesen and Tomita, 1981). In about 20% of cases there are tumours in other endocrine organs, notably the parathyroids and the pituitary, a condition referred to as multiple endocrine adenomatosis, type 1 (see review by Newsome, 1974).

At endoscopy peptic ulcers, often multiple, may be present in unusual sites such as beyond the duodenal bulb and in the oesophagus, or occur after previous gastric surgery. In cases where the diagnosis is made earlier there may be erosive duodenitis only (Regan and Malagelada, 1978). Prominent rugal folds in the stomach are usual and indistinguishable from the appearance in Menetrier's disease.

Histologically, a number of abnormalities can be present. Full thickness biopsy of the body mucosa shows marked thickening due to glandular hyperplasia resulting from a proliferation of parietal cells (Fig. 8.22). There may be an extension of the specialized glandular epithelium into the antrum so that virtually the entire gastric mucosa is of fundal type (Neuberger *et al.*, 1972). Foveolae are normal and there is no associated inflammation. Duodenal biopsies show features of non-specific duodenitis (Section 11.1.2) in which gastric metaplasia of the surface epithelium is a prominent feature (James, 1964; Parrish and Rawlins, 1965). Proliferation of Grimelius positive enterochromaffin-like (ECL) cells in the stomach has been described (Bordi *et al.*, 1974), and occurs in other conditions where there is a raised serum gastrin (Section 8.1.2(b)).

In antral G cell hyperplasia (Fig. 8.23) the endocrine cells are larger than

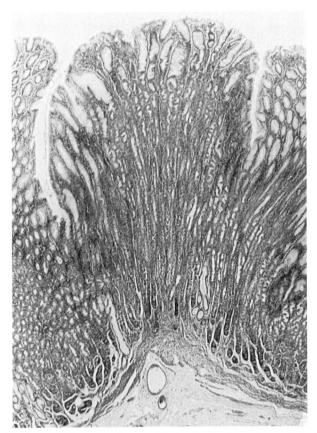

Fig. 8.22   Zollinger-Ellison syndrome. Markedly thickened gastric body mucosa due to hyperplasia of parietal cells. HE × 27.

normal and greatly increased, sometimes forming small clusters or microadenomas (Polak *et al.*, 1972). In the Zollinger-Ellison syndrome there are normal or decreased numbers of antral gastrin cells associated with a gastrinoma (Arnold *et al.*, 1982).

Hyperplasia of gastrin cells in the gastric antrum can occur in a number of other clinical settings. These include pernicious anaemia (Creutzfeldt *et al.*, 1971; Strickland *et al.*, 1971), acromegaly (Pearse and Bussolati, 1970), hyperparathyroidism, after truncal or selective proximal vagotomy, and with a retained gastric antrum following a Polya partial gastrectomy (Pohl *et al.*, 1972). As a group, duodenal ulcer patients have normal numbers of gastrin cells (Creutzfeldt *et al.*, 1976; Piris and Whitehead, 1979) although sub-groups with hypergastrinaemia have been described (Calam *et al.*, 1979).

8.2.2   Menetrier's disease

Since the original description in 1888 of what Menetrier called 'polyadénomes en nappe' (see Palmer, 1968), approximately 300 cases

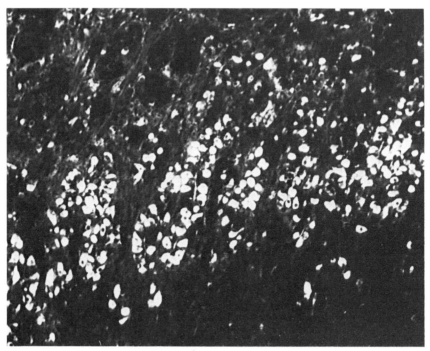

Fig. 8.23   Indirect immunofluorescence staining for gastrin showing hyperplasia of G-type cells in the antrum, × 250.

have been reported of this enigmatic disorder (Cooper and Chadwick, 1981). Pathologically it is characterized by enormous thickening of gastric folds which may additionally have a nodular or polypoid appearance. Body mucosa is affected particularly along the greater curve (Kenney *et al.*, 1954), with or without antral sparing (Olmsted *et al.*, 1976) and the involved areas typically resemble cerebral convolutions. The common clinical symptoms associated with these changes are epigastric pain, which is often food-related, weight loss, vomiting and diarrhoea. Occasionally presentation is with haematemesis or melaena. Acid-secretion studies show that the majority of patients have hypo- or achlorhydria (Scharschmidt, 1977) and there is a non-selective loss of plasma proteins into the gastric lumen, often resulting in a low serum albumin and sometimes associated with peripheral oedema. At endoscopy superficial erosions may be present, and large amounts of viscous mucus coat the enlarged folds. The latter are not effaced even after maximal air insufflation.

Histological examination shows that the mucosa is markedly thickened due to extreme elongation and tortuosity of the gastric pits and to a lesser extent to elongation of the glands (Fig. 8.24). This is most prominent in the apical regions of the gastric folds, and between the folds the mucosa may be of normal thickness. The body glands may contain a relatively normal distribution of specialized cells but usually there is a variable replacement by mucin-secreting cells (Fig. 8.25). Cysts lined by similar epithelium often develop, most commonly in the basal portion of the glandular layer (Fig. 8.26) but sometimes higher. These cysts may penetrate the muscularis mucosae. Inflammation is usually not a conspicuous feature but polymorphs may be present in the lamina propria and within the lumen of glands. Lymphoid follicles can be prominent. There is often considerable oedema particularly in the superficial part of the mucosa. Thickening and fragmentation of the muscularis mucosae occurs and prolongations of this smooth muscle extend between the glands and may reach the surface. Intestinal metaplasia is unusual. Because of the enormous thickening of the mucosa it is obvious that normal sized biopsies will only contain hyperplastic surface and foveolar epithelium, which although consistent with a diagnosis of Menetrier's disease can also result from other disorders such as infiltrating carcinoma or lymphoma. Thus a full thickness mucosal biopsy obtained either at laparotomy or by an electrosurgical snare at endoscopy (Bjork *et al.*, 1977) is essential to make the diagnosis.

The nature of Menetrier's disease is unknown and its aetiology may be multifactorial. The few cases reported in children have been of a self-limited illness and the presence of a peripheral eosinophilia in the majority has suggested the possibility of an allergic reaction in this age group (Chouraqui *et al.*, 1981). The natural history of the disease in adults is unclear since the majority of cases in the literature have had a gastric resection soon after diagnosis. Occasional examples of spontaneous remission have been reported in which protein loss from the stomach has stopped, and this has been accompanied by histological transition to an atrophic gastritis (Frank and Kern, 1967; Berenson *et al.*, 1976).

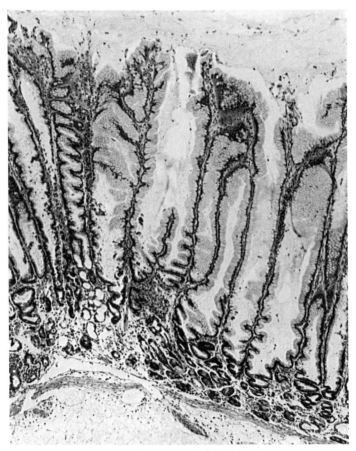

Fig. 8.24   Menetrier's disease. There is marked elongation and some tortuosity of gastric foveolae. HE × 71.

Fig. 8.25   Menetrier's disease. The mucosa is markedly thickened and many of deeper glands are lined by mucin-secreting epithelium and show variable cystic dilatation. HE × 27.

Fig. 8.26   Menetrier's disease. There is marked cystic dilatation of glands deep in the mucosa. HE × 10.

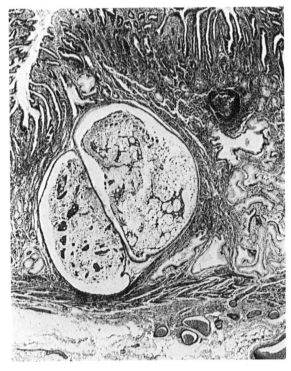

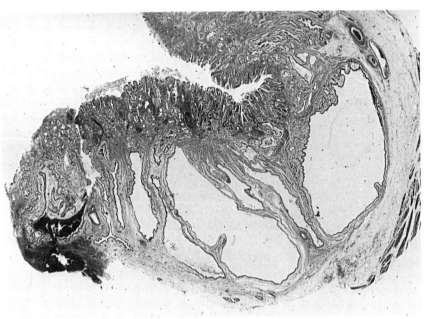

A major point of controversy has related to the cancer risk in Menetrier's disease (Chusid *et al.*, 1964). In several cases the finding of thickened gastric folds at endoscopy, or after radiological examination at the time of diagnosis of gastric cancer, has been attributed to Menetrier's disease, but adequate histological confirmation has been lacking and it is more likely that an infiltrating carcinoma has given rise to this appearance secondarily. As well as this, gastric resection soon after the diagnosis of Menetrier's disease has been the usual method of treatment in the past so that in these instances any possible cancer risk could not be assessed. In a few cases, however, gastric cancer has been detected several years after the diagnosis of Menetrier's disease (van Loewenthal *et al.*, 1960; Chusid *et al.*, 1964; Wood *et al.*, 1983). Because of this it would seem advisable to advocate regular endoscopic follow-up with gastric biopsy in the increasing proportion of patients who are managed medically.

References

Ali, M., Weinstein, J., Biempica, L. *et al.* (1980), Cronkhite-Canada syndrome: report of a case with bacteriologic, immunologic, and electron microscopic studies. *Gastroenterology*, **79**, 731–736.

Andrew, A. (1982), The APUD concept: where has it led us? *Br. Med. Bull.*, **38**, 221–225.

Arnold, R., Hülst, M. V., Neuhof, Ch. *et al.* (1982), Antral gastrin-producing G-cells and somatostatin-producing D-cells in different states of gastric acid secretion. *Gut*, **23**, 285–291.

Beacham, C. H., Shields, H. M., Raffensperger, E. C. and Enterline, H. T. (1978), Juvenile and adenomatous gastrointestinal polyposis. *Dig. Dis.*, **23**, 1137–1143.

Berenson, M. M., Sannella, J. and Freston, J. W. (1976), Menetrier's disease. Serial morphological, secretory, and serological observations. *Gastroenterology*, **70**, 257–263.

Bjork, J. T., Geenen, J. E., Soergel, K. H. *et al.* (1977), Endoscopic evaluation of large gastric folds. A comparison of biopsy techniques. *Gastrointest. Endosc.*, **24**, 22–23.

Bordi, C., Cocconi, G., Togni, R. *et al.* (1974), Gastric endocrine cell proliferation. Association with Zollinger-Ellison syndrome. *Arch. Pathol.*, **98**, 274–278.

Bordi, C., Senatore, S. and Missale, G. (1976), Gastric carcinoid following gastrojejunostomy. *Dig. Dis.*, **21**, 667–671.

Burt, R. W., Berenson, M. M., Lee, R. G. *et al.* (1984), Upper gastrointestinal polyps in Gardner's syndrome. *Gastroenterology*, **86**, 295–301.

Calam, J., Krasner, N. and Haqqani, M. (1982), Extensive gastrointestinal damage following a saline emetic. *Dig. Dis. Sci.*, **27**, 936–940.

Calam, J., Taylor, I. L., Dockray, G. J. *et al.* (1979), Sub-group of duodenal ulcer patients with familial G-cell hyperfunction and hyperpepsinogenaemia I. *Gut.*, **20**, 935 (abstract).

Chejfec, G. and Gould, V. E. (1977), Malignant gastric neuroendocrinomas. Ultrastructural and biochemical characterization of their secretory activity. *Hum. Pathol.*, **8**, 443–440.

Chouraqui, J. P., Roy, C. C., Brochu, P. *et al.* (1981), Menetrier's disease in children: report of a patient and review of sixteen other cases. *Gastroenterology*, **80**, 1042–1047.

Christodoulopoulos, J. B. and Klotz, A. P. (1961), Carcinoid syndrome with primary carcinoid tumour of the stomach. *Gastroenterology*, **40**, 429–440.

Chusid, E. L., Hirsch, R. L. and Colcher, H. (1964), Spectrum of hypertrophic gastropathy. Giant rugal folds, polyposis, and carcinoma of the stomach – case report and review of the literature. *Arch. Int. Med.*, **114**, 621–628.

Cochet, B., Carrel, J., Desbaillets, L. and Widgren, S. (1979), Peutz-Jeghers syndrome associated with gastrointestinal carcinoma. Report of two cases in a family. *Gut*, **20**, 169–175.

Cooper, B. T. and Chadwick, V. S. (1981), Menetrier's disease. In *Gastroenterology 1 Foregut* (ed. J. H. Baron and F. G. Moody), Butterworths, London, pp. 141–191.

Creutzfeldt, W., Arnold, R., Creutzfeldt, C. *et al.* (1971), Gastrin and G-cells in the antral mucosa of patients with pernicious anaemia, acromegaly and hyperparathyroidism and in a Zollinger-Ellison tumour of the pancreas. *Eur. J. Clin. Invest.*, **1**, 461–479.

Creutzfeldt, W., Arnold, R., Creutzfeldt, C. and Track, N. S. (1976), Mucosal gastrin concentration, molecular forms of gastrin, number and ultrastructure of G-cells in patients with duodenal ulcer. *Gut*, **17**, 745–754.

Cronkhite, L. W. Jr. and Canada, W. J. (1955), Generalized gastrointestinal polyposis. An unusual syndrome of polyposis, pigmentation, alopecia and onychotrophia. *N. Engl. J. Med.*, **252**, 1011–1015.

Dirschmid, K., Walser, J. and Hügel, H. (1984), Pseudomalignant erosion in hyperplastic gastric polyps. *Cancer*, **54**, 2290–2293.

Dodds, W. J., Schulte, W. J., Hensley, G. T. and Hogan, W. J. (1972), Peutz-Jeghers syndrome and gastrointestinal malignancy. *Am. J. Roentgenol.*, **115**, 374–377.

Dutta, S. K. and Costa, B. S. (1979), Umbilicated gastric polyposis: an indicator of metastatic gastric tumor. *Am. J. Gastroenterol.*, **71**, 598–604.

Eichenberger, P., Hammer, B., Gloor, F. *et al.* (1980), Gardner's syndrome with glandular cysts of the fundic mucosa. *Endoscopy*, **12**, 63–67.

Elster, K. (1974), A new approach to the classification of gastric polyps. *Endoscopy*, **6**, 44–47.

Elster, K. (1976), Histologic classification of gastric polyps. In *Current Topics in Pathology*, Vol. 63, *Pathology of the Gastro-Intestinal Tract* (ed. B. C. Morson), Springer-Verlag, Berlin, pp. 77–93.

Elster, K., Eidt, H., Ottenjann, R. *et al.* (1977), Drusenkorperzysten, eine polypoide lasion der magenschleimhaut. *Dtsch. Med. Wochenschr.*, **102**, 183–187.

Frank, B. W. and Kern, F. Jr. (1967), Menetrier's disease. Spontaneous metamorphosis of giant hypertrophy of the gastric mucosa to atrophic gastritis. *Gastroenterology*, **53**, 953–960.

Friesen, S. R. and Tomita, T. (1981), Pseudo-Zollinger-Ellison syndrome. Hypergastrinemia, hyperchlorhydria without tumor. *Ann. Surg.*, **194**, 481–493.

Goldman, H., French, S. and Burbige, E. (1981), Kulchitsky cell hyperplasia and multiple metastasizing carcinoids of the stomach. *Cancer*, **47**, 2620–2626.

Goldman, R. L. and Friedman, N. B. (1967), Neurogenic nature of so-called inflammatory fibroid polyps of the stomach. *Cancer*, **20**, 134–143.

Goodman, Z. D., Yardley, J. H. and Milligan, F. D. (1979), Pathogenesis of colonic polyps in multiple juvenile polyposis. Report of a case associated with gastric polyps and carcinoma of the rectum. *Cancer*, **43**, 1906–1913.

Gregory, R. A., Grossman, M. I., Tracy, H. J. and Bentley, P. H. (1967), Nature of the gastric secretagogue in Zollinger-Ellison tumours. *Lancet*, **ii**, 543–544.

Grigioni, W. F., Alampi, G., Martinelli, G. and Piccaluga, A. (1981), Atypical juvenile polyposis. *Histopathology*, **5**, 361–376.

Gueller, R. and Haddad, J. K. (1975), Gastric carcinoids simulating benign polyps. Two cases diagnosed by endoscopic biopsy. *Gastrointest. Endosc.*, **21**, 153–155.

Hajdu, S. I., Winawer, S. J. and Myers, W. P. L. (1974), Carcinoid tumors. A study of 204 cases. *Am. J. Clin. Pathol.*, **61**, 521–528.

Helwig, E. B. and Ranier, A. (1952), Inflammatory fibroid polyps of the stomach. *Am. J. Pathol.*, **28**, 535–536.

Hirata, Y., Sakamoto, N., Yamamoto, H. *et al.* (1976), Gastric carcinoid with ectopic production of ACTH and β-MSH. *Cancer*, **37**, 377–385.

Hodges, J. R., Isaacson, P. and Wright, R. (1981), Diffuse enterochromaffin-like (ECL) cell hyperplasia and multiple gastric carcinoids: a complication of pernicious anaemia. *Gut*, **22**, 237–241.

Iida, M., Yao, T., Watanabe, H. *et al.* (1980), Spontaneous disappearance of fundic gland polyposis: report of three cases. *Gastroenterology*, **79**, 725–728.

Ikeda, K., Sannohe, Y. and Murayama, H. (1981), A case of Cronkhite-Canada syndrome developing after hemi-colectomy. *Endoscopy*, **13**, 251–253.

James, A. H. (1964), Gastric epithelium in the duodenum. *Gut*, **5**, 285–294.

Jarnum, S. and Jensen, H. (1966), Diffuse gastrointestinal polyposis with ectodermal changes. A case with severe malabsorption and enteric loss of plasma proteins and electrolytes. *Gastroenterology*, **50**, 107–118.

Järvinen, H. and Franssila, K. O. (1984), Familial juvenile polyposis coli; increased risk of colorectal cancer. *Gut*, **25**, 792–800.

Johansen, A. (1979), Elevated early gastric carcinoma. Differential diagnosis as regards adenomatous polyps. *Pathol. Res. Pract.*, **164**, 316–330.

Johnston, M. M., Vosburgh, J. W., Wiens, A. T. and Walsh, G. C. (1962), Gastrointestinal polyposis associated with alopecia, pigmentation and atrophy of the fingernails and toenails. *Ann. Intern. Med.*, **56**, 935–940.

Johnstone, J. M. and Morson, B. C. (1978), Inflammatory fibroid polyp of the gastrointestinal tract. *Histopathology*, **2**, 349–361.

Jones, R. A. and Dawson, I. M. P. (1977), Morphology and staining patterns of endocrine cell tumours in the gut, pancreas and bronchus and their possible significance. *Histopathology*, **1**, 137–150.

Kamiya, T., Morishita, T., Asakura, H. *et al.* (1982), Long-term follow-up study on gastric adenoma and its relation to gastric protruded carcinoma. *Cancer*, **50**, 2496–2503.

Kenney, F. D., Dockerty, M. B. and Waugh, J. M. (1954), Giant hypertrophy of gastric mucosa. A clinical and pathological study. *Cancer*, **7**, 671–681.

Kindbloom, L., Angervall, L., Santesson, B. and Selander, S. (1977), Cronkhite-Canada syndrome. *Cancer*, **39**, 2651–2657.

Kozuka, S., Masamoto, K., Suzuki, S. *et al.* (1977), Histogenetic types and size of polypoid lesions in the stomach, with special reference to cancerous change. *Gann*, **68**, 267–274.

Larsson, L-I., Rehfeld, J.F., Stockbrügger, R. *et al.* (1973), Antropyloric gastrinoma associated with pancreatic nesidioblastosis and proliferation of islets. *Virchows Arch. Pathol. Anat. A*, **360**, 305–314.

Larsson, L-I., Rehfeld, J. F., Stockbrügger, R. *et al.* (1978), Mixed endocrine gastric tumors associated with hypergastrinemia of antral origin. *Am. J. Pathol.*, **93**, 53–68.

Lattes, R. and Grossi, C. (1956), Carcinoid tumors of the stomach. *Cancer*, **9**, 698–711.

Lemmer, K. E. (1942), Carcinoid tumors of the stomach. *Surgery*, **12**, 378–382.

Marcus, F. S., Friedman, M. A., Callen, P. W. *et al.* (1980), Successful therapy of an ACTH-producing gastric carcinoid APUD tumor: report of a case and review of the literature. *Cancer*, **46**, 1263–1269.

Menetrier, P. (1888), Des polyadénomes gastriques et de leurs rapport avec le cancer de l'estomac. *Arch. Physiol. Norm. Pathol.* **1**, 32–55, 236–262.

Ming, S-C. (1977), The classification and significance of gastric polyps. In *The Gastrointestinal Tract* (eds J. H. Yardley, B. C. Morson and M. R. Abell), Williams and Wilkins, Baltimore, pp. 149–175.

Ming, S-C. and Goldman, H. (1965), Gastric polyps; a histogenetic classification and its relation to carcinoma. *Cancer*, **18**, 721–726.

Morgan, J. E., Kaiser, C. W., Johnson, W. *et al.* (1983), Gastric carcinoid (gastrinoma) associated with achlorhydria (pernicious anaemia). *Cancer*, **51**, 2332–2340.

Mori, K., Shinya, H. and Wolff, W. I. (1971), Polypoid reparative mucosal proliferation at the site of a healed gastric ulcer: sequential gastroscopic, radiological and histological observation. *Gastroenterology*, **61**, 523–529.

Morson, B. C. (1955), Gastric polyps composed of intestinal epithelium. *Br. J. Cancer*, **9**, 550–557.

Muto, T. and Oota, K. (1970), Polypogenesis of gastric mucosa. *Gann*, **61**, 435–442.

Nakamura, T. (1970), Pathohistologische einteilung der magenpolypen mit spezifischer betrachtung ihrer malignen entartung. *Chirurg*, **41**, 122–130.

Neuburger, Ph., Lewin, M. and Bonfils, S. (1972), Parietal and chief cell populations in four cases of the Zollinger-Ellison syndrome. *Gastroenterology*, **63**, 937–942.

Newsome, H. H. (1974), Multiple endocrine adenomatosis. *Surg. Clin. N. Am.*, **54**, 387–393.

Oberhelman, H. A. Jr. (1972), Excisional therapy for ulcerogenic tumors of the duodenum. Long-term results. *Arch. Surg.*, **104**, 447–453.

Olmsted, W. W., Cooper, P. H. and Madewell, J. E. (1976), Involvement of the gastric antrum in Menetrier's disease. *Am. J. Roentgenol.*, **126**, 524–529.

Palmer, E. D. (1968), What Menetrier really said. *Gastrointest. Endosc.*, **15**, 83–90; 109.

Parrish, J. A. and Rawlins, D. C. (1965), Intestinal mucosa in the Zollinger-Ellison syndrome. *Gut*, **6**, 286–289.

Pearse, A. G. E. and Bussolati, G. (1970), Immunofluorescence studies of the distribution of gastrin cells in different clinical states. *Gut*, **11**, 646–648.

Pestana, C., Beahrs, O. H. and Woolner, L. B. (1963), Multiple (seven) carcinoids of the stomach. Report of case. *Mayo Clin. Proc.*, **38**, 453–456.

Piris, J. and Whitehead, R. (1979), Gastrin cells and fasting gastrin levels in duodenal ulcer patients: a quantitative study based on multiple biopsy specimens. *J. Clin. Pathol.*, **32**, 171–178.

Plachta, A. and Speer, F. D. (1957), Gastric polyps and their relationship to carcinoma of the stomach; review of literature and report of 65 cases. *Am. J. Gastroenterol.*, **28**, 160–175.

Pohl, W., Flachsenberg, E. and Elster, K. (1972), Endoscopic-bioptical diagnosis of antral mucosa within the duodenal stump. *Endoscopy*, **4**, 162–163.

Polak, J. M., Stagg, B. and Pearse, A. G. E. (1972), Two types of Zollinger-Ellison syndrome: immunofluorescent, cytochemical and ultrastructural studies of the antral and pancreatic gastrin cells in different clinical states. *Gut*, **13**, 501–512.

Ranzi, T., Castagnone, D., Velio, P. *et al.* (1981), Gastric and duodenal polyps in familial polyposis coli. *Gut*, **22**, 363–367.

Ray, M. B., Geboes, K., Callea, F. and Desmet, V. J. (1982), Alpha-1-antitrypsin immunoreactivity in gastric carcinoid. *Histopathology*, **6**, 289–297.

Regan, P. T. and Malagelada, J-R. (1978), A reappraisal of clinical, roentgenographic, and endoscopic features of the Zollinger-Ellison syndrome. *Mayo Clin. Proc.*, **53**, 19–23.

Remmele, W. and Kolb, E. F. (1978), Malignant transformation of hyperplasiogenic polyps of the stomach. *Endoscopy*, **10**, 63–65.

Rogers, L. W. and Murphy, R. C. (1979), Gastric carcinoid and gastric carcinoma. Morphologic correlates of survival. *Am. J. Surg. Pathol.*, **3**, 195–202.

Rösch, W. (1980), Epidemiology, pathogenesis, diagnosis and treatment of benign gastric tumours. *Front. Gastrointest. Res.*, **6**, 167–184.

Royston, C. M. S., Brew, D. St. J., Garnham, J. R. *et al.* (1972), The Zollinger-Ellison syndrome due to an infiltrating tumour of the stomach. *Gut*, **13**, 638–642.

Rubin, W. (1973), A fine structural characterization of the proliferated endocrine cells in atrophic gastric mucosa. *Am. J. Pathol.*, **70**, 109–118.

Russo, A., Buffa, R., Grasso, G. *et al.* (1980), Gastric carcinoma and diffuse G-cell hyperplasia associated with chronic atrophic gastritis. Endoscopic detection and removal. *Digestion*, **20**, 416–419.

Ruymann, F. B. (1969), Juvenile polyps with cachexia. Report of an infant and comparison with Cronkhite-Canada syndrome in adults. *Gastroenterology*, **57**, 431–438.

Scharschmidt, B. F. (1977), The natural history of hypertrophic gastropathy (Menetrier's disease). Report of a case with 16 year follow-up and review of 120 cases from the literature. *Am. J. Med.*, **63**, 644–652.

Seifert, E. and Elster, K. (1977), Carcinoids of the stomach. Report of two cases. *Am. J. Gastroenterol.*, **68**, 372–378.

Sipponen, P., Laxen, F. and Seppala, K. (1983), Cystic 'hamartomatous' gastric polyps: a disorder of oxyntic glands. *Histopathology*, **7**, 729–737.

Solcia, E., Capella, C. and Vassallo, G. (1970), Endocrine cells of the stomach and pancreas in states of gastric hypersecretion. *Rendic. R. Gastroenterol.*, **2**, 147–158.

Stemper, T. J., Kent, T. H. and Summers, R. W. (1975), Juvenile polyposis and gastrointestinal carcinoma. A study of a kindred. *Ann. Intern. Med.*, **83**, 639–646.

Strickland, R. G., Bhathal, P. S., Korman, M. G. and Hansky, J. (1971), Serum gastrin and the antral mucosa in atrophic gastritis. *Br. Med. J.*, **4**, 451–453.

Sugano, H., Nakamura, K. and Takagi, K. (1971), An atypical epithelium of the stomach. A clinico-pathological entity. In *Early Gastric Cancer*, Gann Monograph on Cancer Research, 11 (ed. T. Murakami), University of Tokyo Press, Tokyo, pp. 257–269.

Sweeney, E. C. and McDonnell, L. (1980), Atypical gastric carcinoids. *Histopathology*, **4**, 215–224.

Tatsuta, M., Okuda, S., Tamura, H. and Taniguchi, H. (1981), Polyps in the acid-secreting area of the stomach. *Gastrointest. Endosc.*, **27**, 145–149.

Tomasulo, J. (1971), Gastric polyps: histologic types and their relationship to gastric carcinoma. *Cancer*, **27**, 1346–1355.

Ureles, A. L., Alschibaja, T., Lodico, D. and Stabins, S. J. (1961), Idiopathic eosinophilic infiltration of the gastrointestinal tract, diffuse and circumscribed. *Am. J. Med.*, **30**, 899–909.

Utsunomiya, J., Gocho, H., Miyanaga, T. *et al.* (1975), Peutz-Jeghers syndrome: its natural course and management. *Johns Hopkins Med. J.*, **136**, 71–82.

Utsunomiya, J., Maki, T., Iwama, T. *et al.* (1974), Gastric lesion of familial polyposis coli. *Cancer*, **34**, 745–754.

van Loewenthal, M., Steinitz, H. and Friedlander, E. (1960), Gastritis hypertrophica gigantea und Magenkarzinom. *Gastroenterologia*, **93**, 133–144.

Vanek, J. (1949), Gastric submucosal granuloma with eosinophilic infiltration. *Am. J. Pathol.*, **25**, 397–411.

Watanabe, A., Nagashima, H., Motoi, M. and Ogawa, K. (1979), Familial juvenile polyposis of the stomach. *Gastroenterology*, **77**, 148–151.

Watanabe, H., Enjoji, M., Yao, T. and Ohsato, K. (1978), Gastric lesions in familial adenomatosis coli. Their incidence and histologic analysis. *Hum. Pathol.*, **9**, 269–283.

Wilander, E., Grimelius, L., Lundqvist, G. and Skoog, V. (1979), Polypeptide hormones in argentaffin and argyrophil gastroduodenal endocrine tumors. *Am. J. Pathol.*, **96**, 519–530.

Wilander, E., Portela-Gomes, G., Grimelius, L. and Westermark, P. (1977), Argentaffin and argyrophil reactions of human gastrointestinal carcinoids. *Gastroenterology*, **73**, 733–736.

Williams, C. B., Goldblatt, M. and Delaney, P. V. (1982), 'Top and tail endoscopy' and follow-up in Peutz-Jeghers syndrome. *Endoscopy*, **14**, 82–84.

Williams, R. M. (1981), An ultrastructural study of a jejunal inflammatory fibroid polyp. *Histopathology*, **5**, 193–203.

Wood, G. M., Bates, C., Brown, R. C. and Losowsky, M. S. (1983), Intramucosal carcinoma of the gastric antrum complicating Menetrier's disease. *J. Clin. Pathol.*, **36**, 1071–1075.

Zollinger, R. M. and Ellison, E. H. (1955), Primary peptic ulceration of the jejunum associated with islet cell tumors of the pancreas. *Ann. Surg.*, **142**, 709–728.

9 Epithelial dysplasia, adenocarcinoma and other tumours of the stomach

This chapter will consider precancerous changes affecting the gastric epithelium, gastric adenocarcinoma and other benign and malignant neoplasms of the stomach, except for those already discussed in Chapter 8.

9.1 Epithelial dysplasia

As well as the diagnosis of overt malignancy there is increasing interest in the recognition and significance of precancerous changes in the stomach, for which the term epithelial dysplasia is used. The facility of taking multiple directed biopsies from the stomach provided by flexible endoscopy, particularly from individuals with precancerous conditions; i.e. clinical states associated with a significantly increased risk of cancer such as pernicious anaemia (Section 6.3) or the operated stomach (Section 6.4), has meant that the histopathologist will see appearances which at one end of the spectrum merge into and may be difficult to separate from reactive or hyperplastic epithelial changes, and at the other can be impossible to distinguish from malignancy. The difficulty in recognizing and categorizing these changes is reflected in the number of classifications of gastric epithelial dysplasia which have been proposed (Grundmann, 1975; Ming, 1979; Cuello *et al.*, 1979; Oehlert *et al.*, 1979; Morson *et al.*, 1980; Jass, 1983; Ming *et al.*, 1984). These show points of similarity but also significant differences, notably the inclusion in some, as low grade dysplasia, of epithelial changes associated with regeneration, and commonly seen in active gastritis or related to benign peptic ulcers (Figs 6.28, 6.30 and 9.1). As well as this, some classifications have been based on biopsy material whereas others have been retrospective. In the latter, mucosal changes have been assessed in resection specimens, with significance attached to appearances present in cancer-related mucosa and absent in benign conditions. Dysplasia has usually been described in metaplastic epithelium (Fig. 9.2) but can also occur in non-metaplastic

166

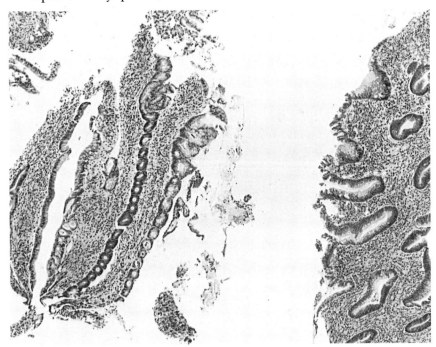

Fig. 9.1   Regenerative and hyperplastic changes of the foveolar epithelium in biopsies from a peptic ulcer. HE × 60.

foveolar epithelium (Fig. 9.3). It may be present in a flat mucosa or as a circumscribed elevation or polyp. Its distribution can be focal, multifocal or diffuse.

The best characterized type is that occurring in adenomas (Section 8.2.1(a)), uncommon lesions which in surgical series have frequently been large, but following the widespread use of endoscopy have been more often detected as small, sessile, slightly elevated, lobulated polyps often with a central depression. Because of the atypical features present histologically they were referred to as borderline or group III lesions (Nagayo, 1971) or as atypical epithelium (Sugano *et al.*, 1971) but are now widely accepted as representing small adenomas. These lesions characteristically consist of deeply stained glands often with a regular tubular pattern and lined by epithelium composed of tall columnar cells with basal rod-shaped nuclei crowded together. Small amounts of mucin, usually sulphated, are often present at the apex of the cell, and Paneth cells and goblet cells may also be seen. The dysplastic epithelium is located in the superficial part of the mucosa and deep to it are metaplastic or mucous-lined glands which are frequently cystically dilated (Fig. 9.4).

The junction of dysplastic and non-dysplastic epithelium is sharp (Fig. 9.5). With increasing degrees of dysplasia the nuclei become oval or rounded, vary in size, are often not so deeply stained, and contain prominent nucleoli. Nuclear stratification and loss of polarity develop and increased numbers of mitoses are present. Mucin secretion is minimal or absent and Paneth cells disappear. Associated with these cytological changes and abnormalities of differentiation there is increasing disorganization of the architecture of the glands with bunching and a back-to-back arrangement. Carcinoma is diagnosed when dysplastic cells are seen to have penetrated the basal membrane of the pits/glands and

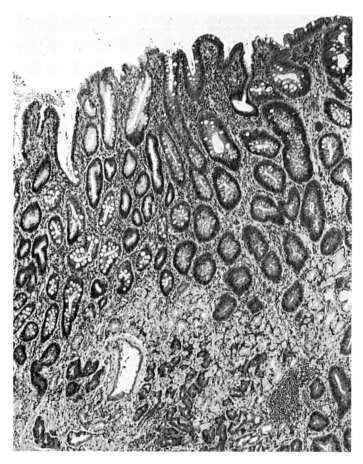

Fig. 9.2 Non-dysplastic glands and surface epithelium showing intestinal metaplasia (left) contrast with metaplastic epithelium in which there is minor epithelial dysplasia (right). Gastric body glands are seen in the lower half of the mucosa. HE × 60.

spilled into the lamina propria (Fig. 9.6). This may be obvious, but there are circumstances where the distinction between severe degrees of dysplasia and a well differentiated tubular or papillary carcinoma is impossible (Fig. 9.7). The expression carcinoma *in situ* is not a suitable one in this situation since the distinctive criteria for this diagnosis in a multi-layered squamous epithelium such as that of the skin or cervix cannot be applied to the single layered epithelium of the stomach, where focal invasion may occur unpredictably. Follow-up of adenomas has demonstrated their malignant potential with carcinomas mostly occurring in tumours over 2 cm in diameter (Kamiya *et al.*, 1982). These lesions should be removed if feasible.

Another type of dysplasia described in endoscopic biopsies from flat mucosa (Cuello *et al.*, 1979) and mucosa adjacent to poorly differentiated

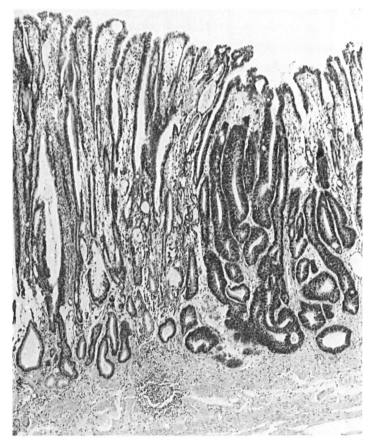

Fig. 9.3 Severe epithelial dysplasia in non-metaplastic foveolar epithelium. HE × 60.

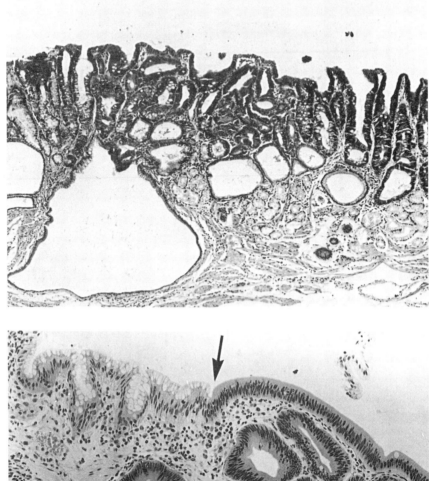

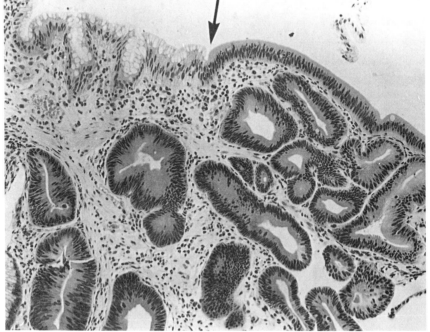

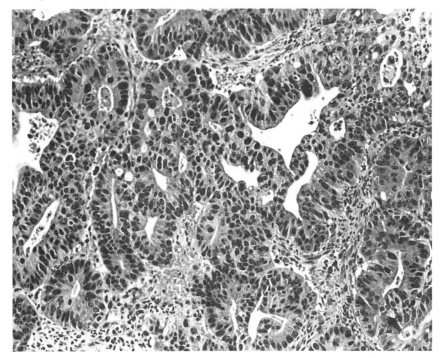

Fig. 9.6   Marked cytological and architectural atypia with budding and a back-to-back arrangement of glands. In places neoplastic cells have spread into the lamina propria. This was one of several biopsies from a papillary lesion close to the cardia, the others showing features of an adenoma. HE × 150.

carcinomas of intestinal type in resection specimens (Jass, 1983) consists of irregularly branched crypts which can vary in size and shape and which show serration and cystic change. The lining cells are columnar with eosinophilic or pale cytoplasm and enlarged round or ovoid nuclei. They contain variable amounts of acid mucin (Fig. 9.8). Goblet cells are sparse or absent and Paneth cells are usually not seen. This form of dysplasia has been termed 'hyperplastic' (Cuello *et al.*, 1979) or Type II (Jass, 1983). In my experience this type of change is rare and I have not encountered it in biopsies.

The types of dysplasia described are associated with the development of, or accompany, intestinal type gastric cancers. Dysplasia does not

Fig. 9.4   Adenoma. Moderately dysplastic epithelium with metaplastic features overlies mucous glands some of which are cystically dilated. HE × 60.
Fig. 9.5   Adenoma. Dysplastic and non-dysplastic epithelium in a biopsy from a sessile polyp in antrum. Note sharp transition on surface (arrowed). HE × 135.

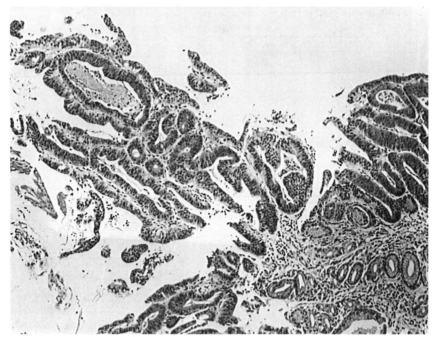

Fig. 9.7 Severely dysplastic epithelium with a papillary configuration in places. A definite diagnosis of carcinoma is not possible in this case, but was made subsequently following repeat endoscopy and biopsy. HE × 80.

appear to play a prominent role, or may be a more subtle change, in the development of diffuse type carcinoma. However some authors have described proliferation and rounding up of mucin-containing cells with loss of polarity of the nuclei in the neck region of the gastric glands and a change in the nature of their mucin which becomes alcianophilic (Schlake and Grundmann, 1979; Oehlert, 1984).

Although in its widest sense dysplasia can be used to describe any cellular deviation from the normal, to have any clinical value its use in pathological reports should be restricted to those abnormalities which appear to represent a neoplastic alteration of the epithelial cells. There are situations of course where it is not possible in small biopsy samples to be certain whether the changes are the result of florid hyperplasia or dysplasia (Section 9.2.2), and a report should state this together with a request for further specimens. As well as this, obviously dysplastic epithelium may itself be malignant and associated with direct invasion into surrounding tissues, although this may not be apparent in the biopsies. When these groups of cases are excluded, which can only be done retrospectively, dysplasia is not a common lesion in my experience.

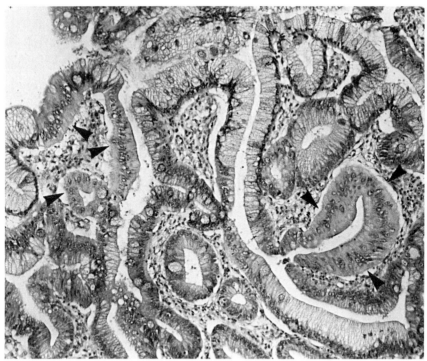

Fig. 9.8 Hyperplastic dysplasia (Type II dysplasia). Focal areas of epithelium composed of tall cells with eosinophilic cytoplasm and enlarged nuclei (arrowed) are interspersed or bud off from epithelium in which there is an incomplete type of intestinal metaplasia. HE × 108.

Serck-Hanssen *et al.* (1984) in Oslo found lesions which they graded as severe dysplasia in 1.8% of gastric biopsy material from patients with varying degrees of chronic gastritis and atrophy in a three-year period. Of the 40 patients with a diagnosis of severe dysplasia on biopsy, 16 had no focal lesion at endoscopy, ten had polyps, nine had a 'tumour' and in five there were ulcers. Twenty-two cancers have been diagnosed on follow-up (of up to five years) in this group, although at least 13 of them represented either cancer-associated dysplasia or well differentiated adenocarcinoma at the time of the initial examination.

Some studies have suggested that in a proportion of cases epithelial dysplasia may spontaneously regress (Oehlert *et al.*, 1979), and regression has also been observed in the operated stomach following bile diversion (Watt *et al.*, 1983). Although this is a possibility, more likely explanations would seem to be either related to sampling, particularly where no visible endoscopic lesion has been present, or to overdiagnosis of hyperplastic changes. There is clearly a need for more prospective studies, particularly in high-risk groups, to clarify and unify the pathological criteria of dysplasia in the stomach and to determine its natural evolution and thus its clinical implications.

9.2   Adenocarcinoma

Gastric adenocarcinoma is of major importance world-wide as a cause of death from malignant disease. In the United Kingdom it results in approximately 12 500 deaths per year making it the third commonest fatal malignancy after carcinoma of the bronchus and large bowel. In the USA, where it is the sixth most common cause of cancer mortality, there are some 14 000 deaths per year, whereas in Japan there are approximately 50 000 deaths per year, accounting for over 30% of deaths from malignant neoplasms in that country. The dismal prognosis associated with advanced gastric cancer has prompted increasing efforts to diagnose cancer at a curable stage and flexible endoscopy of the upper gastrointestinal tract has played the major role in this.

9.2.1   Early gastric cancer

Early gastric cancer is the term used to describe cancer limited to the mucosa or which has extended into the submucosa, irrespective of lymph node metastasis. The word early does not refer to a chronological stage in the genesis of cancer but is used to mean gastric cancer which can be cured (Murakami, 1971). In fact study of these cancers has shown that some may remain confined to the superficial layers for several years, although expanding laterally to a considerable degree, whereas others penetrate the gastric wall rapidly and can invade into the submucosa when they are of the order of 3–5 mm in diameter (Oohara et al., 1982; Kodama et al., 1983). Early gastric cancer (egc) is categorized on the basis of its macroscopic appearance into three main types, polypoid (type I), superficial (type II) and excavated or ulcer-associated (type III), with the superficial group divided into elevated (IIa), flat (IIb) and depressed (IIc) subtypes. The definitive diagnosis of egc is dependent of course on histological examination following resection or excision. The Japanese with their extensive use of endoscopy and wide experience of the often subtle changes which characterize many of these lesions now diagnose up to 30% of gastric cancers at this 'early' stage (Kawai, 1971) and increasing numbers of egcs are being detected outside Japan.

In many series type IIc has been the most frequent macroscopic type of pure form (Nakamura et al., 1967) but combination types, particularly those associated with ulcers (e.g. III + IIc, IIc + III), are also very common. Protruding lesions (types I and IIa), which have a higher tendency than other types to be multiple, have formed a considerable proportion of some European series (Grigioni *et al.*, 1980; Johansen, 1981). There is no obvious relationship between the different macroscopic types of egc and the histological appearances, except that protruding lesions are nearly always well-differentiated glandular adenocarcinomas. Congo red dye spraying at endoscopy has shown that polypoid egcs are associated with minimal or absent acid secretion whereas with ulcerated lesions the acid-secreting area, visible as blue-black discoloration of the dye, is generally large (Tatsuta *et al.*, 1979). An important study by Nakamura and colleagues (1967) of egcs of different size showed that erosion or ulceration occurred significantly more frequently in the larger tumours, suggesting that ulceration was a secondary event and not the predisposing lesion in which cancer subsequently developed. Like benign ulcers, malignant ulcers can heal on medical therapy and this was observed in over 70% of cases in one study (Sakita *et al.*, 1971).

9.2.2   Biopsy appearances of gastric cancer

The range of biopsy appearances of 'early' gastric cancer do not differ from those seen in tissue taken from advanced gastric cancer. With material from type I and IIa egcs the appearances of a well-differentiated adenocarcinoma may be difficult to distinguish from severe dysplasia in an adenoma, and macroscopically these lesions can be identical. The diagnosis of early gastric cancers cannot be made in biopsies even if cancer cells are restricted to the superficial half of the mucosa, since the biopsy is only a sample and not necessarily representative. However, the finding of malignant tissue coupled with characteristic endoscopic appearances may allow a presumptive diagnosis to be made. This is important because close collaboration between endoscopist, pathologist and surgeon in such cases is essential to ensure that a subsequent resection specimen is received fresh from the operating theatre in order that the subtle changes often present are not overlooked (Mochizuki, 1971).

A major source of gastric biopsy material comes from ulcerated lesions. The majority of gastric cancers are ulcerated and at endoscopy malignancy is suggested by features such as an irregular raised margin, club-like thickening and fusion of radiating mucosal folds and nodularity of the ulcer base. However a significant proportion of ulcers lacking these appearances and thought to be benign endoscopically have been shown to be malignant when biopsied. As has been mentioned partial or complete healing of an ulcer with medical treatment cannot be equated with a benign course as this sequence is common with malignant lesions. As well as this the site of origin of benign ulcers and cancer in the stomach is similar, so that localization of an ulcer has no differential diagnostic significance (Evans and Cleary, 1979). It follows therefore that all ulcerated lesions seen at endoscopy, even when appearing to be healing, should be systematically biopsied. Six to ten or more samples should be taken from around the inner margin and from the base if the ulcer is shallow (Hatfield *et al.*, 1975; Dekker and Tytgat, 1977; Graham *et al.*, 1982). Cytological specimens should also be obtained (Section 14.2.2).

In the majority of cases the diagnosis of malignancy is straightforward and some of the variety of appearances are illustrated (Figs 9.9, 9.10 and 9.11). The routine use of a mucin stain is particularly valuable for detecting or confirming the presence of solitary or small clusters of cancer cells of signet ring cell type in the lamina propria (Fig. 9.12). These are variably PAS or alcian blue positive (Yamashiro *et al.*, 1977), therefore a

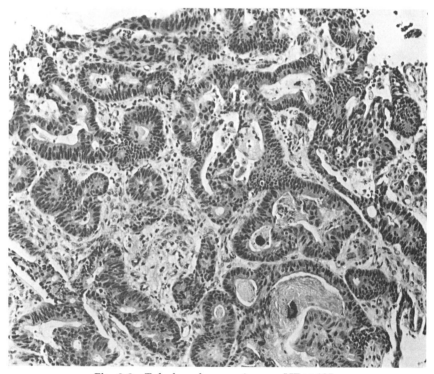

Fig. 9.9   Tubular adenocarcinoma. HE × 135.

Fig. 9.10   Adenocarcinoma with papillary structure. Clear cell appearance in many areas. HE × 132.

Fig. 9.11   Reticulated pattern with strands of poorly differentiated adenocarcinoma infiltrating between gastric glands. HE × 60.

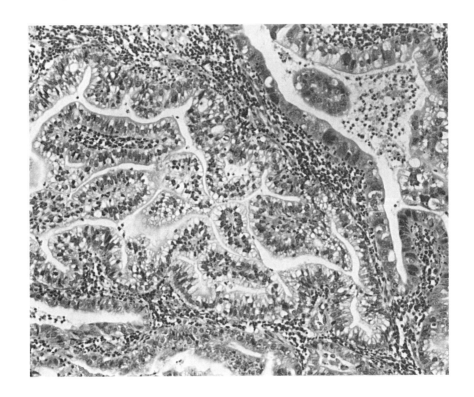

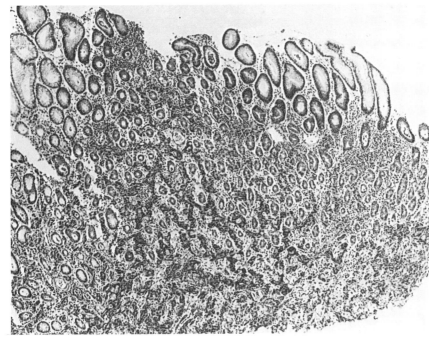

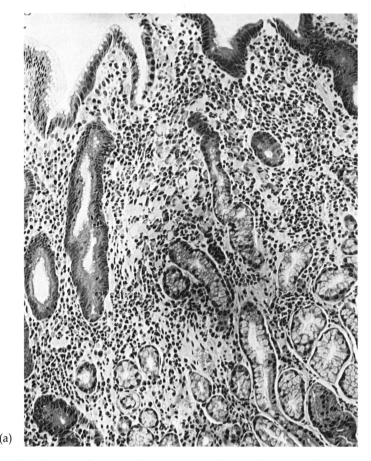

(a)

Fig. 9.12   (a) A small group of signet-ring cells is only just visible and could be easily overlooked. HE × 150.

combined stain is best suited for their detection. It is important to distinguish these cells from the foamy macrophages seen in xanthelasma (Section 13.4).

The difficulties in distinguishing severe degrees of epithelial dysplasia from carcinoma have been discussed above (Section 9.1). In practice a much commoner problem is the distinction of florid regenerative changes occurring for example at the edge of a healing peptic ulcer, from dysplasia or carcinoma. Irregular branching of glands may occur in this situation, with immaturity of the epithelial cells which show an increased nuclear/cytoplasmic ratio, nuclear hyperchromatism and increased numbers of mitoses (Figs 9.13 to 9.16). Glands may become entrapped within hyperplastic and distorted elements of the muscularis mucosae resulting in a

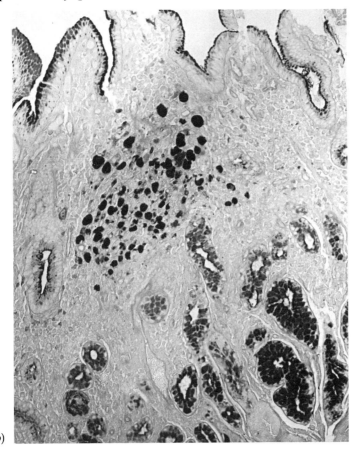

(b)

(b) The same field stained for mucin clearly delineates the malignant cells. PAS/
AB × 150.

spurious appearance of invasion. Usually these changes are associated
with a prominent polymorphonuclear leucocytic infiltration of the epithelium and lamina propria although active inflammation may also be
seen in association with cancer. Biopsies from erosions may also show
features which can be misinterpreted as malignant (Isaacson, 1982).
Closely packed glands which vary in size are lined by cells with swollen
cytoplasm which often contain hyperchromatic nuclei. They are present
in an eosinophilic background matrix with erosion of the surface epithelium. Unlike malignant glands they merge into adjacent more obvious
regenerative mucosa (Figs 7.1 and 7.2).

There are other circumstances where careful interpretation is necessary. Exuberant granulation tissue examined at low power mimics an

infiltrating microglandular carcinoma (Figs 9.17 and 9.18). This contrasts with the appearance of malignant cells associated with granulation tissue (Fig. 9.19). Biopsies from the base of a penetrating peptic ulcer may contain pancreatic (Fig. 9.20) or liver tissue and particularly in the latter case the cords of liver cells can superficially resemble carcinoma (Figs 9.21 and 9.22). Marked epithelial atypia associated with glandular crowding and distortion and misinterpreted as carcinoma has also been reported in biopsies from the margins of peptic ulcers which have developed as a complication of arterial infusion chemotherapy used to treat primary hepatic carcinoma and liver metastases (Weidner *et al.*, 1983). Collections of mucous cells shed from the mucosa in the region of ulcers or erosions may resemble signet ring carcinoma cells but show as well varying degrees of autolysis (Figs 9.23 and 9.24). The possibility of misinterpreting changes due to crushing has been mentioned earlier (Section 1.4 and Figs 1.3 and 1.4).

The presence in biopsies of conspicuous numbers of so-called Russell bodies in plasma cells (Fig. 9.25) has been shown to correlate with the

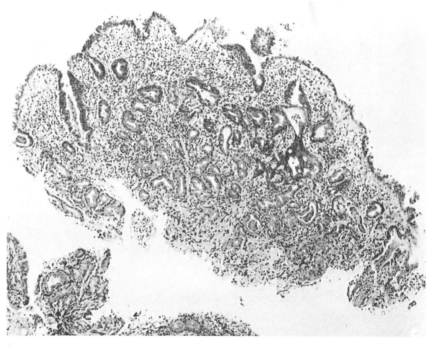

Fig. 9.13 Biopsy from edge of antral lesser curve ulcer. Hyperchromasia of foveolar and surface epithelium and an area where there is considerable architectural distortion. HE × 67.

presence of carcinoma (Johansen and Sikjar, 1977) as has the finding of gram-positive filamentous intertwining organisms (Fig. 9.26). The latter have been observed in a proportion of ulcerated intestinal type gastric cancers but not in the base of benign peptic ulcers (Mickalek *et al.*, 1982). If these features are noted in material which does not contain malignant tissue it suggests a sampling error and indicates the need for repeat biopsies.

Examination of multiple biopsies from a lesion gives a much better overview of the pattern of the changes present and their significance

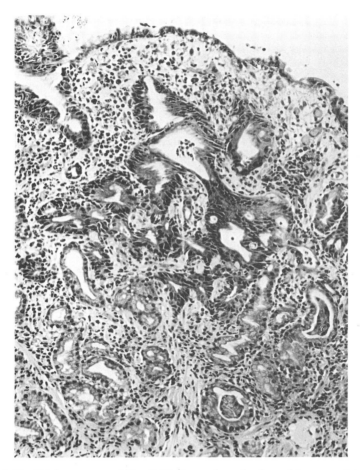

Fig. 9.14   Higher power of Fig. 9.13 shows foveolar branching associated with hyperchromasia of the epithelium. Note large numbers of polymorphs in the lamina propria and epithelium. Appearances were considered to warrant repeat endoscopy with multiple biopsies – no carcinoma present. HE × 150.

than interpretation based on a single or few samples, and potentially worrying features seen in an individual piece of tissue assume less sinister connotations when taken in conjunction with appearances in the others. Of course even when multiple biopsies have been taken, malignant change can be present in only one piece, but this is a sampling problem and the appearances of malignancy are nearly always distinctive. There will however be cases in which it is not possible to be certain whether the process is malignant or reactive and where repeat endoscopy and biopsy is necessary. With increasing experience this situation will only occur occasionally but it hardly needs to be said that if there is any doubt at all this course has to be followed. Another endoscopic examination is at most a nuisance, an unwarranted gastrectomy is a disaster.

9.2.3   Classification of adenocarcinoma

The WHO classification of papillary, tubular, mucinous and signet-ring cell types (Oota and Sobin, 1977) is satisfactory for reporting gastric cancer in biopsies. Sometimes a mixture of patterns can be present. Those

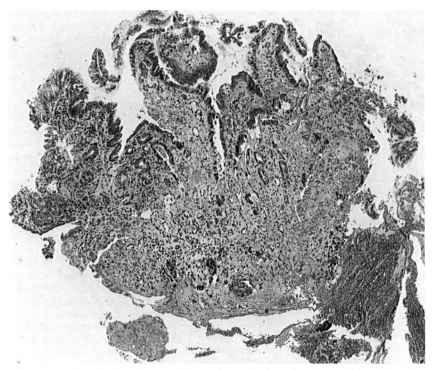

Fig. 9.15   Gastric ulcer biopsy. Blood clot and ulcer slough on right. HE × 60.

classifications dividing gastric cancer into intestinal and diffuse types (Lauren, 1965) or expanding and infiltrative types (Ming, 1977) are not applicable to biopsies, since they are largely dependent on an assessment of the growth patterns of gastric cancer, which can only be determined in resection specimens.

9.3   Adenosquamous and squamous cell carcinoma

Occasional cases of adenosquamous carcinoma have been reported in the stomach (Straus *et al.*, 1969; Mingazzini *et al.*, 1983) mostly in the distal

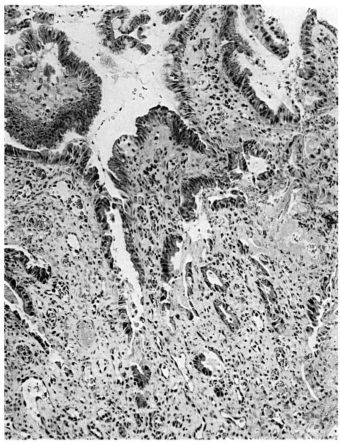

Fig. 9.16 Detail of Fig. 9.15 shows marked regenerative changes of the surface and glandular epithelium on a background of granulation tissue. The fragmented appearance of the glands and the cytological changes give a superficial impression of carcinoma. HE × 126.

half. They consist of varying proportions of glandular and squamous neoplastic tissue (Fig. 9.27). Pure squamous cell carcinomas are very rare and a glandular component is often present when such tumours are extensively sampled following resection (Straus *et al.*, 1969). They have been described as a complication of gastric involvement in tertiary syphilis (Vaughan *et al.*, 1977) and were observed in two patients following long-term cyclophosphamide therapy (McLoughlin *et al.*, 1980).

9.4   Gastric lymphomas

Primary lymphomas make up about 2% of malignant tumours of the stomach and are the commonest non-epithelial malignancy. The stomach

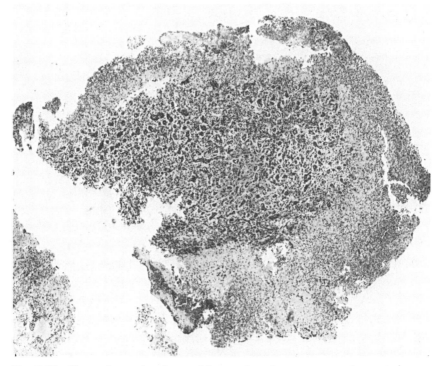

Fig. 9.17   Biopsy from ulcer base with pseudo-acinar structures beneath slough on surface. HE × 48.

Fig. 9.18   Detail of Fig. 9.17 shows exuberant granulation tissue with markedly swollen endothelial cells. HE × 375.
Fig. 9.19   Malignant cells with large hyperchromatic nuclei and little cytoplasm are present in granulation tissue. HE × 375.

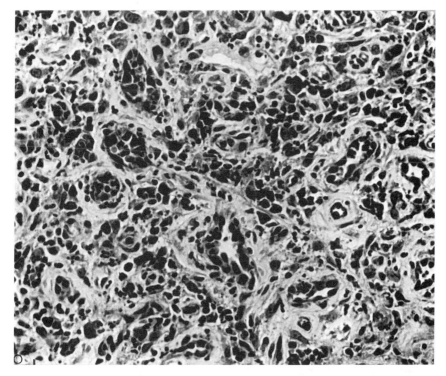

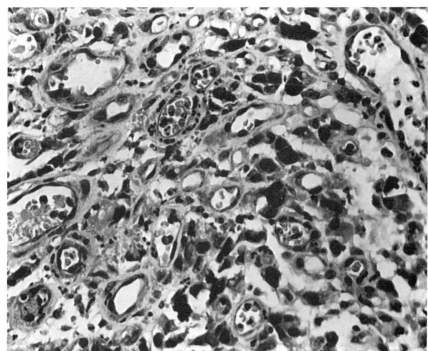

is the major extranodal site for these tumours. The clinical presentation and macroscopic appearances are mostly indistinguishable from gastric carcinoma but the prognosis and management differ.

The classification of gastric lymphomas and the relative proportion of different sub-types presents difficulties which reflect not only the current controversies relating to categorization of lymphomas in general but also the comparative rarity of lymphomas at this site. It is now generally agreed however that primary Hodgkin's disease of the stomach is vanishingly rare. Most of the non-Hodgkin's lymphomas are diffuse but approximately one fifth have a nodular component. Using the Rappaport classification (1966), most have been of diffuse histiocytic type (Lim *et al.*, 1977; Lewin *et al.*, 1978; Brooks and Enterline, 1983*b*), followed by poorly differentiated lymphocytic lymphomas. The Kiel classification (Gerard-Marchant *et al.*, 1974) has given somewhat variable results with different

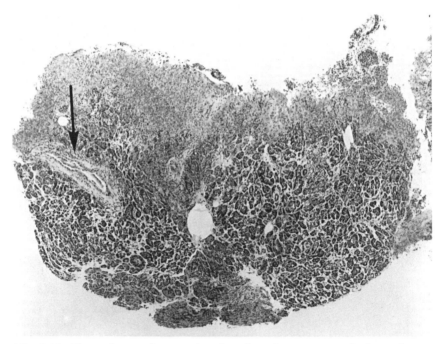

Fig. 9.20 Biopsy from a deep penetrating ulcer shows pancreatic tissue deep to ulcer slough. Pancreatic duct is arrowed. HE × 48.

Fig. 9.21 Cords of liver cells deep to ulcer slough. HE × 62.

Fig. 9.22 Detail of Fig. 9.21 shows bland-appearing cells with plentiful eosinophilic cytoplasm. A higher power showed perinuclear lipofuscin and some canalicular bile. HE × 375.

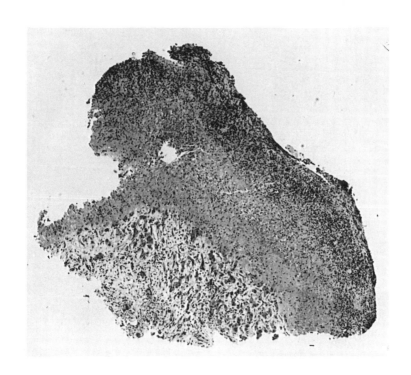

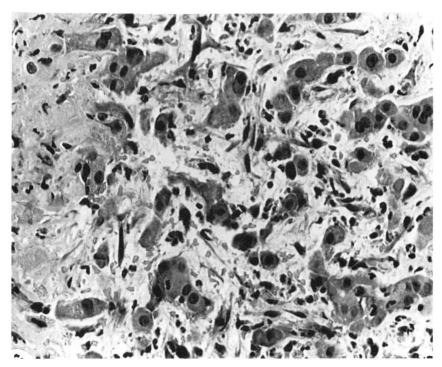

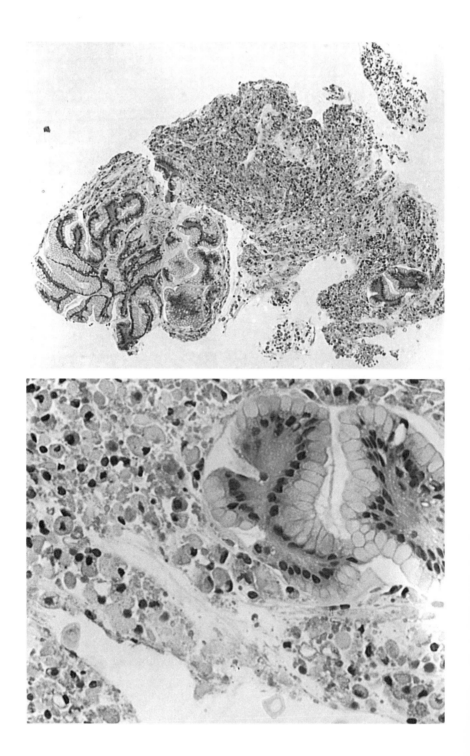

investigators (Isaacson *et al.*, 1979; Heule *et al.*, 1979; Dworkin *et al.*, 1982), but overall, approximately equal numbers of high and low grade tumours in the stomach have been reported. Immunological techniques used to determine surface antigens (Yamanaka *et al.*, 1980) and the presence of intracytoplasmic immunoglobulin (Seo *et al.*, 1982) have suggested that many of these tumours are of B-cell origin. With the Kiel terminology, which will be followed here, most gastric lymphomas are of follicle centre

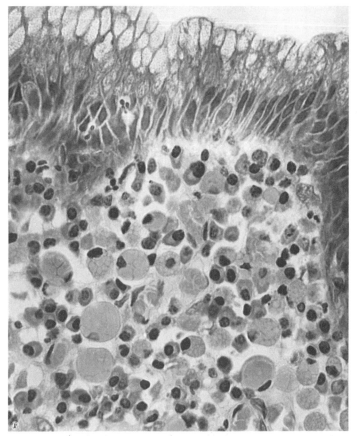

Fig. 9.25 Many plasma cells contain intracellular accumulations of immuno-globulin (so-called Russell bodies). HE × 600.

Fig. 9.23 Superficial fragments of gastric mucosa together with sheets of mucous cells. HE × 75.

Fig. 9.24 Higher power of Fig. 9.23 shows free-lying, rounded mucous cells some with signet-ring cell appearance. However nuclei are pyknotic and many of the cells are undergoing fragmentation. HE × 375.

cell (FCC) origin and contain variable proportions of centrocytes and centroblasts. However some tumours with indistinguishable features from other non-Hodgkin's lymphomas in routine paraffin sections are composed of cells containing lysozyme (muramidase), implying a malignant proliferation of histiocytes (Isaacson et al., 1979; Seo et al., 1982).

A range of appearances may be seen at endoscopy including ulcerated masses, polypoid or nodular bulky growths, or an infiltrative lesion giving rise to rigid, thickened and sometimes giant folds. An unusual volcano-like ulcer crater has been described in some cases (Nelson and Lanza, 1974). In these the histology has been that of an immunoblastic lymphoma (Demling et al., 1982). Any part of the stomach may be affected and multiple lesions may be present (Joseph and Lattes, 1966).

Diagnosis of these tumours by endoscopic biopsy can be achieved in a majority of cases (Nelson and Lanza, 1974; Russo et al., 1978) and this is facilitated when multiple samples or big particle biopsies are taken (Ottenjann et al., 1973). Histologically the appearances are of a dense

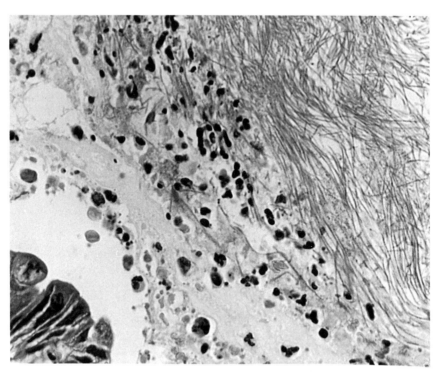

Fig. 9.26 Filamentous organisms and inflammatory débris from ulcer. Cancerous epithelium at bottom left. HE × 600.

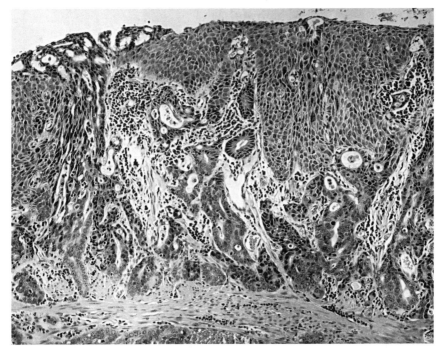

Fig. 9.27 Adenosquamous carcinoma. Mixture of glandular and squamous carcinoma. Plaque-like lesion on anterior wall of mid-stomach. HE × 108.

mucosal infiltrate which separates, compresses or effaces the gastric glands and the surface epithelium when present (Fig. 9.28). Although some variation in cell size is usually present the infiltrate is essentially monomorphous (Fig. 9.29), contrasting with the polymorphous nature of the infiltrate in pseudolymphoma (see below). Focal invasion of glandular epithelium by centrocytes and centroblasts may be seen and Wright and Isaacson (1983) consider this to be pathognomonic of FCC lymphoma. Nuclear size and mitotic rate are also useful features enabling delineation from benign lesions in the majority of cases (Brooks and Enterline, 1983*b*). When muscularis mucosae is included in a biopsy it can be focally destroyed. The two major sources of diagnostic difficulty are firstly the distinction from florid reactive lymphoid hyperplasia, so-called pseudolymphoma (Section 9.4.1), and secondly to distinguish FCC lymphomas in which centroblasts or immunoblasts predominate from undifferentiated carcinoma in which mucin is absent. In this latter situation, immunological staining techniques, examination of plastic-embedded sections, and ultrastructual examination may be necessary. Repeat endoscopy and biopsy may be required to obtain fresh material for diagnosis particularly in centres where non-surgical treatment of gastric lymphoma is carried out.

The prognosis of gastric lymphomas is better overall than for other gastrointestinal lymphomas and carcinomas, and relates best to the stage of disease rather than the histological type (Lewin *et al.*, 1978; Dworkin *et al.*, 1982; Brooks and Enterline, 1983*b*). Thus in one series after surgical resection for cure the overall five-year disease-free survival was 47%. In those without spread to perigastric lymph nodes the survival rate was 78%, decreasing to 29% where local nodal involvement was present (Dworkin *et al.*, 1982). Large tumours have also been associated with a poorer prognosis in some reports (Dworkin *et al.*, 1982; Brooks and Enterline, 1983*b*).

There are few reports of extramedullary plasmacytoma of the stomach although in one series 15 of 51 gastric lymphomas were considered to be of this type (Henry and Farrer-Brown, 1977). This was probably because of the inclusion of tumours showing plasmacytoid differentiation such as lymphoplasmacytic lymphomas (immunocytomas) and follicle centre cell lymphomas. If the term is restricted to tumours in which there is a

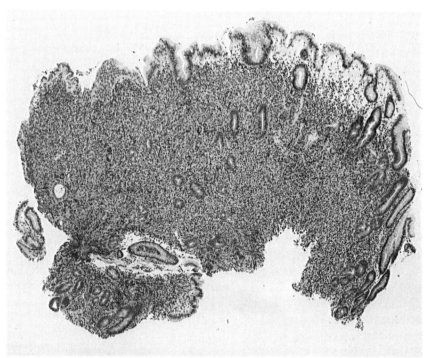

Fig. 9.28 Malignant lymphoma. Diffusely infiltrating tumour separating gastric glands. HE × 48.

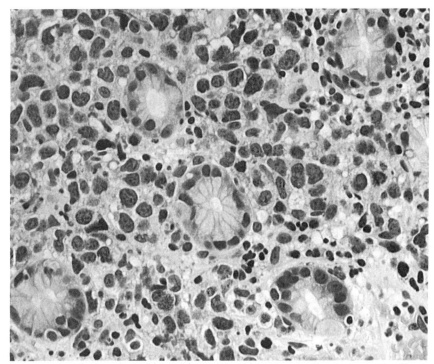

Fig. 9.29   Malignant lymphoma (centroblastic) infiltrating lamina propria. Note preservation of gastric glands. HE × 435.

monotonous proliferation of plasma cells in which varying degrees of pleomorphism are present and in which there is monotypic staining using immunohistochemical techniques (Scott *et al.*, 1978), the prevalence seems to be low. Most lesions have been in the distal stomach and macroscopically are indistinguishable from carcinoma or other lymphoid neoplasms. Paraproteins in the serum and urine are frequently absent.

On rare occasions the stomach can be involved secondarily in multiple myeloma and in one case multiple polyps were seen at gastroscopy (Goeggel-Lamping and Kahn, 1978). Plasmacytoma has to be distinguished from so-called plasma cell granuloma (Soga *et al.*, 1970), an inflammatory condition of unknown cause which can mimic a carcinoma at endoscopy. Histologically there are large numbers of mature plasma cells, but small numbers of lymphocytes and other inflammatory cells are seen in addition. Intra- or extracellular hyaline globules of immunoglobulin are often conspicuous. The polyclonal immunoglobulin pattern demonstrable immunohistochemically confirms the reactive nature of this lesion (Isaacson *et al.*, 1978; Domenichini *et al.*, 1982).

9.4.1   Pseudolymphoma

This lesion, also known as benign or reactive lymphoid hyperplasia, is uncommon, with less than 200 published cases in the English literature. The most frequent macroscopic finding is of an ulcer with overhanging margins, but nodularity and an infiltrative appearance of surrounding tissue may be present. The antrum is the usual site (Hyjek and Kelenyi, 1982). Sometimes there is a mass or plaque without gross ulceration. Although usually single, multiple lesions can occur (Jacobs, 1963). Overall they have a smaller diameter and present in a younger age group than malignant lymphomas, but there is considerable overlap. The diagnosis has nearly always been made from pathological examination of resection specimens or of surgical biopsies, often on the basis of re-analysis of cases where long-term survival militated against the original designation of malignant lymphoma.

Histologically there is an infiltrate of small lymphocytes and the presence of lymphoid aggregates often with germinal centres, together with a variable number of other inflammatory cells including plasma cells, eosinophils and polymorphs (Figs 9.30 and 9.31). Mitoses are few and centrofollicular cells are confined to germinal centres. There is frequently an intimate admixture of fibrous tissue although this is usually more conspicuous in the submucosa than mucosa. Because the distinction between pseudolymphoma and malignant lymphoma in resected material can present real difficulties, it is not surprising that endoscopic biopsy diagnosis has rarely been achieved (Graham, 1982).

The pathogenesis of pseudolymphoma is considered to be an exaggerated response to peptic ulceration, but the changes may persist following healing of the ulcer (Graham, 1982). Although generally considered to be benign there have been recent reports of focal lymphoma associated with a pseudolymphomatous reaction (Brooks and Enterline, 1983a) and of transitional zones between benign reactive follicles and lymphomatous nodules (Heule et al., 1979).

9.5   Smooth muscle tumours

Although smooth muscle tumours of the stomach are often found at autopsy (Meissner, 1944) symptomatic lesions are uncommon, occurring in approximately 0.2% of examinations in one endoscopic series (Lee, 1979). They appear as rounded or ovoid indentations of any part of the stomach and larger lesions show one or more areas of ulceration of the overlying mucosa. Occasional tumours are pedunculated.

Histologically, smooth muscle tumours show a wide range of appearances and variation frequently occurs within individual tumours.

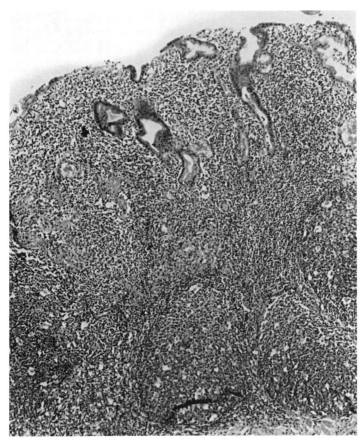

Fig. 9.30 Pseudolymphoma. There is a dense mucosal infiltrate. Several lymphoid follicles are present. HE × 69.

The basic pattern is of easily recognizable spindle-shaped cells with elongated nuclei, arranged in interlacing bundles or with a whorled pattern and often showing nuclear palisading. A variant which occurs with particular frequency in the stomach (Stout, 1962) consists of round or polygonal cells with eosinophilic cytoplasm in which there may be a perinuclear clear area (Fig. 9.32), the latter probably representing fixation artefact (Cornog, 1974). This pattern may occur alone or be a component of a tumour in which spindle cell areas are also present. In the former case the term epithelioid leiomyoma (or leiomyosarcoma) is given (other terms which have been used are bizarre smooth muscle tumour and leiomyoblastoma). The criteria applied in resection specimens to predict the behaviour of spindle cell tumours have been increasing degrees of pleomorphism and a high mitotic count. Those used for tumours with an epithelioid pattern include decreasing size of cells resulting from loss of cytoplasm, angulation and hyperchromatism of nuclei, and variation of morphology from area to area (Appelman and Helwig, 1977). Because of the small size of the samples and the fact that biopsies are often taken from the vicinity of ulcers, where misleading regenerative and degenerative changes in the adjacent tumour cells may be present, the pathologist is wise to confine himself to a diagnosis of 'smooth muscle tumour', unless the tumour is markedly anaplastic.

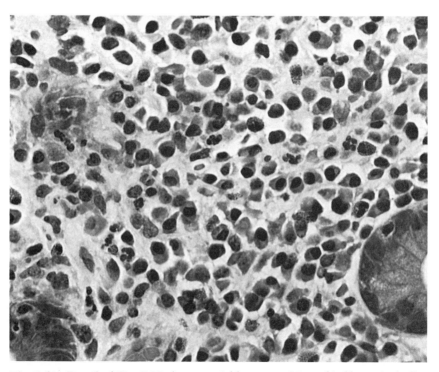

Fig. 9.31 Detail of Fig. 9.30 shows variable composition of infiltrate including plasma cells, eosinophils and polymorphs. HE × 600.

9.6 Vascular tumours

9.6.1 Glomus tumour

Approximately 30 gastric glomus tumours have been reported, most of which have formed sessile masses 1–4 cm in diameter in the distal part of the stomach (Kay *et al.*, 1951; Almagro *et al.*, 1981). They are located in the submucosa, often with extension into the muscularis propria, and ulcera-

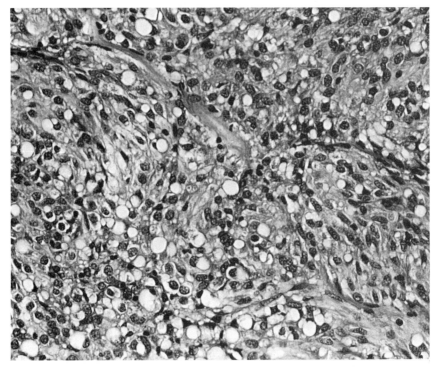

Fig. 9.32   Epithelioid leiomyoma. Most of the cells are round or polygonal and many have vacuolated cytoplasm. HE × 300.

tion of the overlying mucosa results in bleeding, the major clinical symptom. Histologically they are composed of lobules of very uniform cells containing round nuclei with coarsely clumped chromatin and with a moderate amount of eosinophilic cytoplasm (Fig. 9.33). A clear zone partly or completely surrounding the nucleus may be present. Between and within tumour lobules are tortuous and branched thin walled, and generally empty, vascular channels lined by normal endothelium. Ultrastructurally the tumour cells have shown features of smooth muscle or characteristics of pericytes (Osamura *et al.*, 1977). In biopsies the appearances have to be distinguished from those seen in carcinoid tumours and from small cell malignant lymphomas. The organoid pattern, vascularity, lack of staining characteristics associated with endocrine cells, and bland appearance of the tumour cells with few or no mitoses are characteristic, and silver impregnation may demonstrate reticulin fibres surrounding individual cells or small groups of cells. These tumours are benign and their recognition in biopsies will forestall radical surgery, as simple excision is curative.

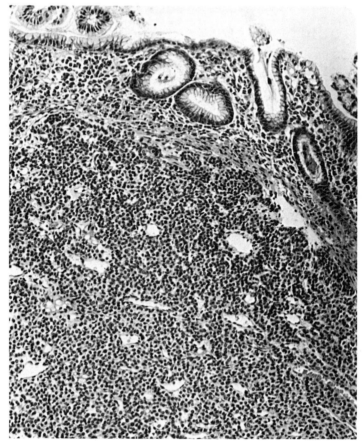

Fig. 9.33   Glomus tumour. Small uniform cells with round nuclei and numerous thin-walled vascular channels. HE × 150.

9.6.2   Kaposi's sarcoma

Kaposi's sarcoma is a rare neoplasm of primitive vasoformative mesenchyme (Akhtar *et al.*, 1984) which in Europe and North America has typically involved the skin of the legs of elderly males and run an indolent course. Visceral involvement is uncommon. Recently however there have been increasing reports in young homosexual males in the USA and elsewhere of an uncommonly severe form of the disease with a widespread distribution of skin lesions, generalized lymphadenopathy and visceral involvement, often associated with unusual opportunistic pathogens (Hymes *et al.*, 1981; Gottlieb *et al.*, 1981). These patients have all had an acquired severe defect in cell mediated immunity, referred to as the acquired immunodeficiency syndrome (AIDS). Kaposi's sarcomas have also arisen in patients with induced immune deficiency, e.g. following renal transplantation (Penn, 1977).

Involvement of the gastrointestinal tract is common in these groups although often asymptomatic. Upper gastrointestinal endoscopy has shown the stomach to be most frequently affected, and a range of appearances can be seen from multiple, purple, maculopapular lesions up to 5 mm in diameter to larger nodular or polypoid areas, or nodules with central umbilication (Ahmed *et al.*, 1975). Histologically, intertwining bundles of atypical spindle-shaped cells are interspersed with endothelial-lined vascular spaces. Extravasated red blood cells, lymphocytes and histiocytes are present (Figs 9.34 and 9.35). The visceral lesions have

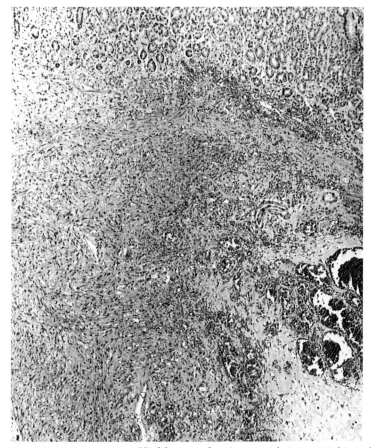

Fig. 9.34   Kaposi's sarcoma. Highly vascular tissue with interstitial interlacing spindle cells. Gastric mucosa above. HE × 60.

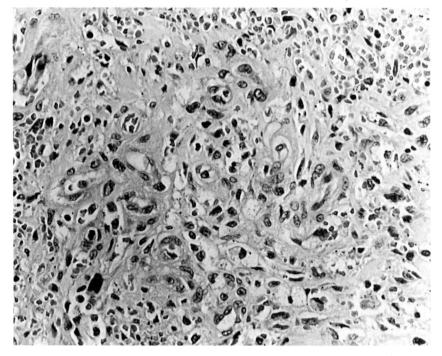

Fig. 9.35   Kaposi's sarcoma. A detail of Fig. 9.34. Note numerous extravasated red blood cells. HE × 375.

responded to chemotherapy, whereas local irradiation is the preferred treatment for disease localized to the skin.

9.7   Other tumours

Occasional examples of primary choriocarcinoma of the stomach have been reported, with a mixture of trophoblastic and carcinoma cells in either the primary tumour or its metastases. In some, chorionic gonadotrophin activity was present in the serum or demonstrated immunohistochemically in the tumour cells (Smith *et al.*, 1980).

Granular cell tumours have occasionally been observed in the stomach (Abdelwahab and Klein, 1983) and may be associated with peptic ulcer symptoms. These well circumscribed, submucosal tumours have been up

Fig. 9.36   Metastatic malignant melanoma. A darkly staining group of cells is present in the lower half of body mucosa. HE × 60.

Fig. 9.37   Large pleomorphic cells containing pigment infiltrate between gastric glands. HE × 600.

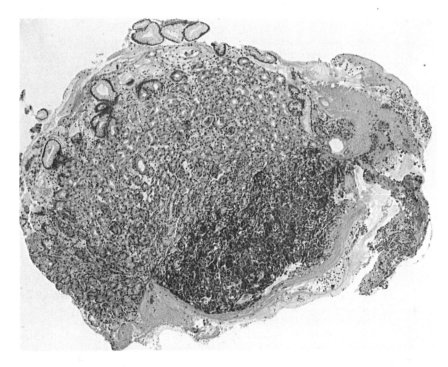

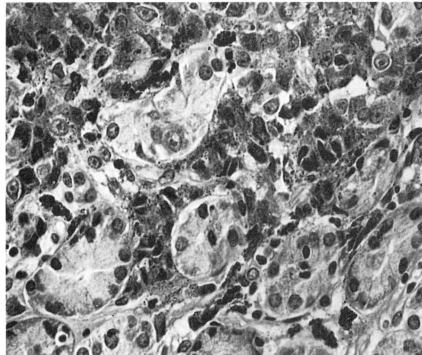

to 4 cm in diameter and may be associated with ulceration of the overlying mucosa.

Metastases to the stomach are uncommon and mostly asymptomatic but may cause haemetemesis, pyloric obstruction or perforation (Menuck and Amberg, 1975; Adams *et al.*, 1983). They have usually been associated with tumours of epithelial origin such as breast (Choi *et al.*, 1964), lung, pancreas, thyroid, prostate and malignant melanoma (Nelson and Lanza, 1978). They can be single or multiple and frequently show central ulceration or umbilication. In biopsies, atypical cells may infiltrate the submucosa and muscularis mucosae, if included, and be seen in the lamina propria, with displacement but preservation of normal appearing gastric glands (Figs 9.36 and 9.37).

References

Abdelwahab, I. F. and Klein, M. J. (1983), Granular cell tumor of the stomach: a case report and review of the literature. *Am. J. Gastroenterol.*, **78**, 71–76.

Adams, H. W., Adkins, J. R. and Rehak, E. M. (1983), Malignant fibrous histiocytoma presenting as a bleeding gastric ulcer. *Am. J. Gastroenterol.*, **78**, 212–213.

Ahmed, N., Nelson, R. S., Goldstein, H. M. and Sinkovics, J. G. (1975), Kaposi's sarcoma of the stomach and duodenum: endoscopic and roentgenologic correlations. *Gastrointest. Endosc.*, **21**, 149–152.

Akhtar, M., Bunuan, H., Ali, M. A. and Godwin, J. T. (1984), Kaposi's sarcoma in renal transplant recipients. Ultrastructural and immunoperoxidase study of four cases. *Cancer*, **53**, 258–266.

Almagro, U. A., Schulte, W. J., Norback, D. H. and Turcotte, J. K. (1981), Glomus tumor of the stomach. Histologic and ultrastructural features. *Am. J. Clin. Pathol.*, **75**, 415–419.

Appelman, H. D. and Helwig, E. B. (1977), Sarcomas of the stomach. *Am. J. Clin. Pathol.*, **67**, 2–10.

Brooks, J. J. and Enterline, H. T. (1983a), Gastric pseudolymphoma. Its three subtypes and relation to lymphoma. *Cancer*, **51**, 476–486.

Brooks, J. J. and Enterline, H. T. (1983b), Primary gastric lymphomas. A clinicopathologic study of 58 cases with long-term follow-up and literature review. *Cancer*, **51**, 701–711.

Choi, S. H., Sheehan, F. R. and Pickren, J. W. (1964), Metastatic involvement of the stomach by breast cancer. *Cancer*, **17**, 791–797.

Cornog, J. L. Jr. (1974), Gastric leiomyoblastoma. A clinical and ultrastructural study. *Cancer*, **34**, 711–719.

Cuello, C., Correa, P., Zarama, G. *et al.* (1979), Histopathology of gastric dysplasias. Correlations with gastric juice chemistry. *Am. J. Surg. Pathol.*, **3**, 491–500.

Dekker, W. and Tytgat, G. N. (1977), Diagnostic accuracy of fiberendoscopy in the detection of upper intestinal malignancy. A follow-up analysis. *Gastroenterology*, **73**, 710–714.

Demling, L., Elster, K., Koch, H. and Rosch, W. (1982), *Endoscopy and Biopsy of*

Esophagus, Stomach and Duodenum. A Color Atlas, W. B. Saunders, Philadelphia, p. 158.

Domenichini, E., Martiarena, H. M. and Rubio, H. H. (1982), Gastric plasma cell granuloma. (Report of a case). *Endoscopy*, **14**, 148–150.

Dworkin, B., Lightdale, C. J., Weingrad, D. N. *et al.* (1982), Primary gastric lymphoma. A review of 50 cases. *Dig. Dis. Sci.*, **27**, 986–992.

Evans, D. M. D. and Cleary, B. K. (1979), The sites of origin of gastric cancers and ulcers in relation to mucosal junctions and the lesser curvature. *Invest. Cell Pathol.*, **2**, 97–117.

Gerard-Marchant, R., Hamlin, I., Lennert, K. *et al.* (1974), Classification of non-Hodgkin's lymphomas. *Lancet*, **ii**, 406–408. (letter).

Goeggel-Lamping, C. and Kahn, S. B. (1978), Gastrointestinal polyposis in multiple myeloma. *J. Am. Med. Assoc.*, **239**, 1786–1787.

Gottlieb, M. S., Schroff, R., Schanker, H. M. *et al.* (1981), *Pneumocystis carinii* pneumonia and mucosal candidiasis in previously healthy homosexual men. Evidence of a new acquired cellular immunodeficiency. *N. Engl. J. Med.*, **305**, 1425–1431.

Graham, D. Y., Schwartz, J. T., Cain, G. D. and Gyorkey, F. (1982), Prospective evaluation of biopsy number in the diagnosis of esophageal and gastric carcinoma. *Gastroenterology*, **82**, 228–231.

Graham, J. R. (1982), Gastric pseudolymphoma developing from chronic gastric ulcer: endoscopic diagnosis and the effect of cimetidine. *Dig. Dis. Sci.*, **27**, 1051–1053. (letter).

Grigioni, W. F., Alampi, G., Bondi, A. *et al.* (1980), Retrospective studies of early gastric cancer in a high incidence area of Italy. *Histopathology*, **4**, 533–545.

Grundmann, E. (1975), Histologic types and possible initial stages in early gastric carcinoma. *Beitr. Pathol.*, **154**, 256–280.

Hatfield, A. R. W., Slavin, G., Segal, A. W. and Levi, A. J. (1975), Importance of the site of endoscopic gastric biopsy in ulcerating lesions of the stomach. *Gut*, **16**, 884–886.

Henry, K. and Farrer-Brown, G. (1977), Primary lymphomas of the gastro-intestinal tract. I. Plasma cell tumours. *Histopathology*, **1**, 53–76.

Heule, B. V., van Kerkem, C. and Heimann, R. (1979), Benign and malignant lymphoid lesions of the stomach. A histological reappraisal in the light of the Kiel classification for non-Hodgkin's lymphomas. *Histopathology*, **3**, 309–320.

Hyjek, E. and Kelenyi, G. (1982), Pseudolymphomas of the stomach: a lesion characterized by progressively transformed germinal centres. *Histopathology*, **6**, 61–68.

Hymes, K. B., Cheung, T., Greene, J. B. *et al.* (1981), Kaposi's sarcoma in homosexual men – a report of eight cases. *Lancet*, **ii**, 598–600.

Isaacson, P. (1982), Biopsy appearances easily mistaken for malignancy in gastrointestinal endoscopy. *Histopathology*, **6**, 377–389.

Isaacson, P., Buchanan, R. and Mepham, B. L. (1978), Plasma cell granuloma of the stomach. *Hum. Pathol.*, **9**, 355–358.

Isaacson, P., Wright, D. H., Judd, M. A. and Mepham, B. L. (1979), Primary gastrointestinal lymphomas. A classification of 66 cases. *Cancer*, **43**, 1805–1819.

Jacobs, D. S. (1963), Primary gastric malignant lymphoma and pseudolymphoma. *Am. J. Clin. Pathol.*, **40**, 379–394.

Jass, J. R. (1983), A classification of gastric dysplasia. *Histopathology*, **7**, 181–193.

Johansen, A. (1981), *Early Gastric Cancer: A Contribution to the Pathology and to Gastric Cancer Histogenesis*. Poul Petri, Copenhagen.

Johansen, A. and Sikjär, B. (1977), The diagnostic significance of Russell bodies in endoscopic gastric biopsies. *Acta Pathol. Microbiol. Scand.*, **85**, 245–250.

Joseph, J. I. and Lattes, R. (1966), Gastric lymphosarcoma. Clinicopathologic analysis of 71 cases and its relation to disseminated lymphosarcoma. *Am. J. Clin. Pathol.*, **45**, 653–669.

Kamiya, T., Morishita, T., Asakura, H. *et al.* (1982), Long-term follow-up study on gastric adenoma and its relation to gastric protruded carcinoma. *Cancer*, **50**, 2496–2503.

Kawai, K. (1971), Diagnosis of early gastric cancer. *Endoscopy*, **3**, 23–27.

Kay, S., Callahan, W. P. Jr., Murray, M. R. *et al.* (1951), Glomus tumors of the stomach. *Cancer*, **4**, 726–736.

Kodama, Y., Inokuchi, K., Soejima, K. *et al.* (1983), Growth patterns and prognosis in early gastric carcinoma. Superficially spreading and penetrating growth types. *Cancer*, **51**, 320–326.

Lauren, P. (1965), The two histological main types of gastric carcinoma: diffuse and so-called intestinal-type carcinoma. An attempt at a histo-clinical classification. *Acta Pathol. Microbiol. Scand.*, **64**, 31–49.

Lee, F. I. (1979), Gastric leiomyoma and leiomyosarcoma – five cases. *Postgrad. Med. J.*, **55**, 575–578.

Lewin, K. J., Ranchod, M. and Dorfman, R. F. (1978), Lymphomas of the gastrointestinal tract. A study of 117 cases presenting with gastrointestinal disease. *Cancer*, **42**, 693–707.

Lim, F. E., Hartman, A. S., Tan, E. G. C. *et al.* (1977), Factors in the prognosis of gastric lymphoma. *Cancer*, **39**, 1715–1720.

McLoughlin, G. A., Cave-Bigley, D. J., Tagore, V. and Kirkham, N. (1980), Cyclophosphamide and pure squamous-cell carcinoma of the stomach. *Br. Med. J.*, **1**, 524.

Meissner, W. A. (1944), Leiomyoma of the stomach. *Arch. Pathol.*, **38**, 207–209.

Menuck, L. S. and Amberg, J. R. (1975), Metastatic disease involving the stomach. *Am. J. Dig. Dis.*, **20**, 903–913.

Michalek, H., Kishaba, T., Ishiharo, M. *et al.* (1982), Filamentous organisms in ulcerated intestinal type carcinoma of the stomach: an aid to biopsy diagnosis. *Histopathology*, **6**, 779–785.

Ming, S-C. (1977), Gastric carcinoma. A pathobiological classification. *Cancer*, **39**, 2475–2485.

Ming, S-C. (1979), Dysplasia of gastric epithelium. *Front. Gastrointest. Res.*, **4**, 164–172.

Ming, S-C., Bajtai, A., Correa, P. *et al.* (1984), Gastric dysplasia. Significance and pathologic criteria. *Cancer*, **54**, 1794–1801.

Mingazzini, P. L., Barsotti, P. and Malchiodi Albedi, F. (1983), Adenosquamous carcinoma of the stomach. *Histopathology*, **7**, 433–443.

Mochizuki, T. (1971), Method for histopathological examination of early gastric cancer. In *Early Gastric Cancer*, Gann Monograph on Cancer Research, 11 (ed. T. Murakami), University of Tokyo Press, Tokyo, pp. 57–65.

Morson, B. C. Sobin, L. H., Grundmann, E. *et al.* (1980), Precancerous conditions and epithelial dysplasia in the stomach. *J. Clin. Pathol.*, **33**, 711–721.

Murakami, T. (1971), Pathomorphological diagnosis. Definition and gross classification of early gastric cancer. In *Early Gastric Cancer*, Gann Monograph on Cancer Research, 11 (ed. T. Murakami), University of Tokyo Press, Tokyo, pp. 53–55.

Nagayo, T. (1971), Histological diagnosis of biopsied gastric mucosae with special reference to that of borderline lesions. In *Early Gastric Cancer*, Gann Monograph on Cancer Research, 11 (ed. T. Murakami), University of Tokyo Press, Tokyo, pp. 245–256.

Nakamura, K., Sugano, H., Takagi, K. and Fuchigami, A. (1967), Histopathological study on early carcinoma of the stomach – some considerations on the ulcer-cancer by analysis of 144 foci of the superficial spreading carcinomas. *Gann*, **58**, 377–387.

Nelson, R. S. and Lanza, F. L. (1974), The endoscopic diagnosis of gastric lymphoma. Gross characteristics and histology. *Gastrointest. Endosc.*, **21**, 66–68.

Nelson, R. S. and Lanza, F. (1978), Malignant melanoma metastatic to the upper gastrointestinal tract. Endoscopic and radiologic correlations, form and evolution of lesions, and value of directed biopsy in diagnosis. *Gastrointest. Endosc.*, **24**, 156–158.

Oehlert, W. (1984), Preneoplastic lesions of the stomach. In *Precursors of Gastric Cancer* (ed. S-C. Ming), Praeger, New York, pp. 73–82.

Oehlert, W., Keller, P., Henke, M. and Strauch, M. (1979), Gastric mucosal dysplasia: what is its clinical significance? *Front. Gastrointest. Res.*, **4**, 173–182.

Oohara, T., Tohma, H., Takezoe, K. *et al.* (1982), Minute gastric cancers less than 5 mm in diameter. *Cancer*, **50**, 801–810.

Oota, K. and Sobin, L. H. (1977), Histological typing of gastric and oesophageal tumours. In *International Histological Classification of Tumours*, no. 18, WHO, Geneva.

Osamura, R. Y., Watanabe, K., Yoneyama, K. and Hayashi, T. (1977), Glomus tumor of the stomach. Light and electron microscopic study with literature review of related tumors. *Acta Pathol. Jpn.*, **27**, 533–539.

Ottenjann, R., Lux, G., Henke, M. and Strauch, M. (1973), Big particle biopsy. *Endoscopy*, **5**, 139–143.

Penn, I. (1977), Kaposi's sarcoma in organ transplant recipients. Report of 20 cases. *Transplantation*, **27**, 8–11.

Rappaport, H. (1966), Tumors of the hematopoietic system. In *Atlas of Tumor Pathology*, section 3, fascicle 8, US Armed Forces Institute of Pathology, Washington, D.C.

Russo, A., Grasso, G., Sanfillipo, G. *et al.* (1978), Gastroscopy and directed biopsy in the diagnosis of primary gastric lymphomas. Report of 16 personal cases. *Tumori*, **64**, 419–427.

Sakita, T., Oguro, Y., Takosu, S. *et al.* (1971), Observations on the healing of ulcerations in early gastric cancer. The life cycle of the malignant ulcer. *Gastroenterology*, **60**, 835–844.

Schlake, W. and Grundmann, E. (1979), Multifocal early gastric cancer of mixed type. *Pathol. Res. Pract.*, **164**, 331–341.

Scott, F. E. T., Dupont, P. A. and Webb, J. (1978), Plasmacytoma of the stomach. Diagnosis with the aid of the immunoperoxidase technique. *Cancer*, **41**, 675–681.

Seo, I. S., Binkley, W. B., Warner, T. F. C. S. and Warfel, K. A. (1982), A combined morphologic and immunologic approach to the diagnosis of gastrointestinal lymphomas. I. Malignant lymphoma of the stomach (a clinicopathologic study of 22 cases). *Cancer*, **49**, 493–501.

Serck-Hanssen, A., Osnes, M. and Myren, J. (1984), Epithelial dysplasia in the stomach: the size of the problem and some preliminary results of a follow-up study. In *Precursors of Gastric Cancer* (ed. S-C. Ming), Praeger, New York, pp. 53–71.

Smith, F. R., Barkin, J. S. and Hensley, G. (1980), Choriocarcinoma of the stomach. *Am. J. Gastroenterol.*, **73**, 45–48.

Soga, J., Saito, K., Suzuki, N. and Sakai, T. (1970), Plasma cell granuloma of the stomach. A report of a case and review of the literature. *Cancer*, **25**, 618–625.

Stout, A. P. (1962), Bizarre smooth muscle tumors of the stomach. *Cancer*, **15**, 400–409.

Straus, R., Heschel, S. and Fortmann, D. J. (1969), Primary adenosquamous carcinoma of the stomach. A case report and review. *Cancer*, **24**, 985–995.

Sugano, H., Nakamura, K. and Takagi, K. (1971), An atypical epithelium of the stomach. A clinico-pathological entity. In *Early Gastric Cancer*, Gann Monograph on Cancer Research, 11 (ed. T. Murakami), University of Tokyo Press, Tokyo, pp. 257–269.

Tatsuta, M., Okuda, S., Taniguchi, H. and Tamura, H. (1979), Gross and histological types of early gastric carcinomas in relation to the acid-secreting area. *Cancer*, **43**, 317–321.

Vaughan, W. P., Straus, F. H. II and Paloyan, D. (1977), Squamous carcinoma of the stomach after luetic linitis plastica. *Gastroenterology*, **72**, 945–948.

Watt, P. C. H., Sloan, J. M., Spencer, A. and Kennedy, T. L. (1983), Histology of the post-operative stomach before and after diversion of bile. *Br. Med. J.*, **287**, 1410–1412.

Weidner, N., Smith, J. G. and LaVanway, J. M. (1983), Peptic ulceration with marked epithelial atypia following hepatic arterial infusion chemotherapy. A lesion initially misinterpreted as carcinoma. *Am. J. Surg. Pathol.*, **3**, 261–268.

Wright, D. H. and Isaacson, P. G. (1983), *Biopsy Pathology of the Lymphoreticular System*, Chapman and Hall, London, pp. 270–273.

Yamanaka, N., Ischii, Y., Koshiba, H. *et al.* (1980), A study of surface markers in gastrointestinal lymphoma. *Gastroenterology*, **79**, 673–677.

Yamashiro, K., Suzuki, H. and Nagayo, T. (1977), Electron microscopic study of signet-ring cells in diffuse carcinoma of the stomach. *Virchows Arch. Pathol. Anat. A.*, **374**, 275–284.

10   The normal duodenal mucosa

10.1   Endoscopic appearances

The duodenum is sub-divided into the bulb, descending, horizontal and ascending parts. The first part, or duodenal bulb, is some 5–6 cm long with its widest diameter just beyond the pylorus and narrowing slightly towards the bend leading into the descending duodenum. Absent or barely visible folds in the bulb contrast with the readily apparent transverse folds (of Kerckring) in the remainder of the duodenum. The papilla of Vater is situated within the descending part at the junction of its medial and posterior walls some 8–10 cm from the pylorus.

10.2   Histology

10.2.1   Mucosa

Although the normal mucosa of the duodenum has a similar composition throughout its length there are differences in morphology, notably relating to villous architecture and Brunner's gland component, between biopsies taken from the proximal and more distal parts. Thus stereomicroscopy of the normal duodenal bulb shows that there is considerable variation in the size and shape of villi, with leaf-shaped forms tending to predominate. Histologically, this is reflected by the villi tending to be shorter, broader and blunter in these areas than distally, and this change can be accentuated when Brunner's glands occupy the lamina propria of the mucosa or in villi overlying lymphoid follicles. In addition there can be considerable variation in villous shape in biopsies from adjacent areas and even within a single biopsy (Fig. 10.1) (Korn and Foroozan, 1974). Villous architecture may also be influenced by the depth of the biopsy, in that absence of the muscularis mucosae can result in an appearance of separated and shortened villi.

The villi are some 0.2–0.5 mm long and are covered by a columnar

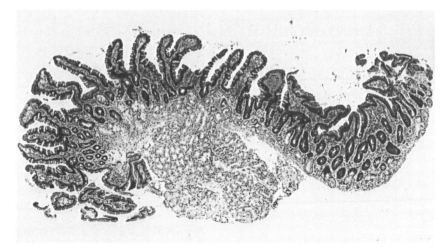

Fig. 10.1 Normal duodenal mucosa. Variation in shape of villi with finger-like and clubbed forms. HE × 40.

epithelium composed predominantly of absorptive cells (enterocytes) with oval, basal nuclei and a prominent brush border which stains positively with PAS, together with scattered goblet cells which contain sialomucins as well as neutral mucins and are alcianophilic when a PAS/AB stain is used. These are most frequent at or near the base of the villi and decrease towards the villous tip (Fig. 10.2). Small numbers of columnar mucin-secreting cells at the tips of some of the villi (Fig. 10.3), so-called gastric metaplasia, are common in biopsies from the first part of the duodenum (Kreuning *et al.*, 1978). The sides of the villi show a series of indentations giving a 'saw tooth' appearance.

The basal layer of the mucosa is some 100–250 µm thick and consists of simple tubular glands or crypts of Leiberkuhn which are continuous with the epithelium of the villi and extend down almost reaching the muscularis mucosae. Cells in the lower two-thirds of the crypt form the proliferative zone of the mucosa, and here there is increased cytoplasmic basophilia and frequent mitotic figures. Lining the glands in this zone are occasional absorptive cells and moderate numbers of goblet cells, and at the bottom of the crypts are the distinctive Paneth cells characterized by the presence in formalin and mercuric-fixed material of large eosinophilic, apical, refractile secretory granules. The granules are less refractile and not so brightly staining in Paneth cells away from the crypt bases. The function of these cells is enigmatic (Sandow and Whitehead, 1979).

The lamina propria occupies the area between the crypts of Lieberkuhn and extends into the villous cores. It consists of loose connective tissue infiltrated by plasma cells, lymphocytes, eosinophils, mast cells and histiocytes together with blood vessels, lymphatics and slips of smooth muscle fibres extending upwards from the muscularis mucosae. Neutrophils are not a feature of the normal lamina propria. The cellular content of the lamina propria shows considerable variation, a feature which has to be borne in mind in the consideration of duodenitis (see Chapter 11). Loosely formed aggregates of lymphocytes and discrete lymphoid follicles are not uncommon in duodenal biopsies (Fig. 10.4). Immunohistochemistry has demonstrated a constant ratio of IgG, IgM and IgA-producing plasma cells with an average ratio of 10 to 2.4 to 1.1 respectively (Kreuning *et al.*, 1978).

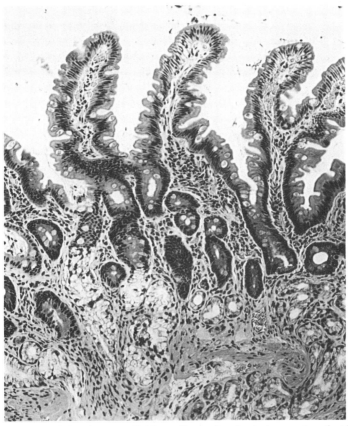

Fig. 10.2   Normal duodenum. Goblet cells predominate in crypt and at base of villi. Note bifid villus at right. HE × 147.

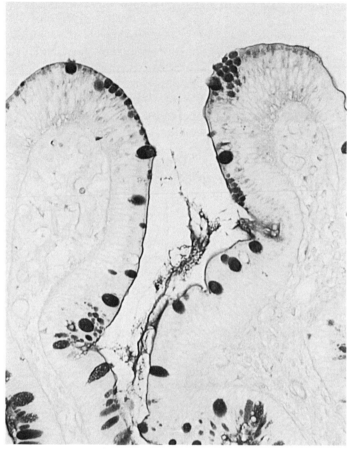

Fig. 10.3   Small numbers of columnar mucous cells at tips of villi. PAS/AB × 250.

10.2.2   Brunner's glands

Brunner's glands are most abundant immediately beyond the pylorus and gradually diminish in number and size distally (Robertson, 1941). They were present in biopsies from the descending duodenum in 34% of a group of asymptomatic volunteers (Kreuning *et al.*, 1978). Occasionally they extend into the pyloric region of the stomach for a short distance. They lie mainly in the submucosa but nearly always reach above the muscularis mucosae as well (Fig. 10.5). They consist of coiled and branched tubulo-alveolar glands lined with mucous cells which are identical in structure and staining properties to the mucous cells of the pyloric glands. Ducts lined by similar cells pass through the muscularis mucosae to open by wide lumina into the crypts of Lieberkuhn (Fig. 10.6).

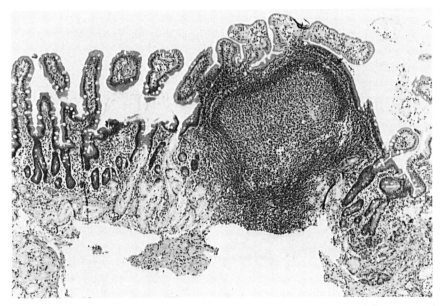

Fig. 10.4 Lymphoid follicle with germinal centre. Distortion and flattening of overlying villi. HE × 65.

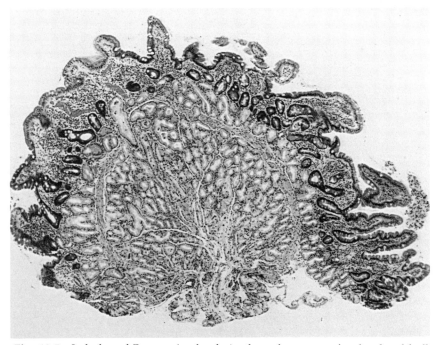

Fig. 10.5 Lobules of Brunner's glands in the submucosa of a duodenal bulb biopsy. Note variation in villous structure. HE × 45.

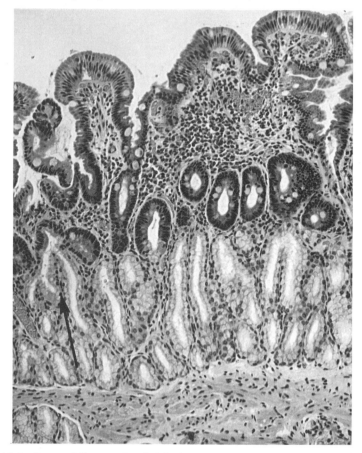

Fig. 10.6 Duct of Brunner's glands in mucosa opening into base of crypts (arrowed). Inflammatory cell infiltrate in lamina propria is within normal limits. HE × 150.

An occasional Paneth cell may be seen in superficial parts of Brunner's glands.

10.2.3   Endocrine cells

Ultrastructural studies, immunocytochemistry and radioimmunoassay have categorized numerous different types of endocrine cell in the duodenal mucosa and Brunner's glands each synthesizing, storing and secreting specific biogenic amines or peptide hormones (Lechago, 1978; O'Briain and Dayal, 1981). Gastrin cells are scattered throughout the mucosal thickness and within Brunner's glands but are outnumbered by those producing cholecystokinin (I cells) and secretin (S cells) which are present in the epithelium of the crypts and villi but have not been described in Brunner's glands. Other cell types identified have been the somatostatin containing D cells, D_1 cells with vasoactive intestinal polypeptide (VIP)-like immunoreactivity, K cells containing gastric inhibitory peptide (GIP), P cells (bombesin), L cells (glucagon-like immunoreactivity) and small numbers of pancreatic polypeptide immunoreactive cells. Three sub-classes of serotonin containing entero-chromaffin cells (EC) are present in the duodenum – EC_n cells, EC_1 cells which also contain substance P, and EC_2 cells containing motilin in addition to serotonin. All these different endocrine cell types are potentially capable of giving rise to tumours of carcinoid morphological type.

References

Korn, E. R. and Foroozan, P. (1974), Endoscopic biopsies of normal duodenal mucosa. *Gastrointest. Endosc.*, **21**, 51–54.

Kreuning, J., Bosman, F. T., Kuiper, G. *et al.* (1978), Gastric and duodenal mucosa in 'healthy' individuals. An endoscopic and histopathological study of 50 volunteers. *J. Clin. Pathol.*, **31**, 69–77.

Lechago, J. (1978), Endocrine cells of the gastrointestinal tract and their pathology. In *Pathology Annual*, vol. 13, part 2 (eds S. C. Sommers and P. P. Rosen), Appleton-Century-Crofts, New York, pp. 329–350.

O'Briain, D. S. and Dayal, Y. (1981), The pathology of the gastrointestinal endocrine cells. In *Diagnostic Immunocytochemistry* (ed. R. A. DeLellis), Masson, New York, pp. 75–109.

Robertson, H. E. (1941), The pathology of Brunner's glands. *Arch. Pathol.*, **31**, 112–130.

Sandow, M. J. and Whitehead, R. (1979), The Paneth cell. *Gut*, **20**, 420–431.

11   Duodenitis

Inflammation of the duodenum may occur in a number of conditions including coeliac disease, Crohn's disease, specific infective and parasitic diseases, and secondary to pathology of the pancreas and biliary tract. Without qualification however the term is used, often prefixed by the words 'chronic non-specific', to describe changes maximal in the duodenal bulb.

11.1   Chronic non-specific duodenitis

Inflammatory changes in the first part of the duodenum may occur alone or in association with a peptic duodenal ulcer when the inflammation is most marked in the immediately adjacent mucosa although it can be widespread within the duodenal bulb. Whether non-specific duodenitis always represents a stage which can lead on to ulceration or alternatively may follow the healing of an ulcer, or whether it is a distinct entity has not been resolved. In earlier studies the clinical diagnosis of duodenitis was based on the history and radiological findings such as coarse folds in the duodenal bulb and rapid transit of contrast material through a spastic duodenum in the absence of an ulcer crater. In addition biopsies were not taken under direct vision (Aronson and Norfleet, 1962; Beck *et al.*, 1965). Radiological appearances however often show poor correlation with changes at endoscopy (Cotton *et al.*, 1973; Nebel *et al.*, 1973) and inflammation in the duodenum is more often patchy than diffuse, so that 'blind' biopsies may fail to sample involved mucosa. A correlation between symptoms of non-ulcer dyspepsia and duodenal inflammation has been found by some investigators (Beck *et al.*, 1965; Cotton *et al.*, 1973; Gelzayd *et al.*, 1973; Thomson *et al.*, 1977) but not by others (Aronson and Norfleet, 1962; Gregg and Garabedian, 1974; Cheli and Aste, 1976; Holdstock *et al.*, 1979). Direct observation of the duodenal mucosa at endoscopy together with the ability to take targeted biopsies has provided the opportunity to diagnose and follow the natural history of duodenitis, its response to treatment and its relationship to peptic ulceration of the duodenum.

214

11.1.1   Endoscopic appearances

A range of appearances may be seen including swelling of the mucosal folds, patchy or diffuse erythema, petechial haemorrhages and erosions. An active or healed ulcer may also be present. Assessment of the changes is carried out with the tip of the endoscope in the pylorus so that trauma to the duodenal mucosa by the instrument is not misinterpreted. Reddening of the mucosa alone does not correlate well with histological duodenitis and may be a vasomotor response in certain individuals, unrelated to inflammation. There is also no doubt that active inflammation may be present in biopsies from a macroscopically normal mucosa.

11.1.2   Histological appearances

The lack of uniformity in defining and classifying inflammatory changes in the duodenum (Classen et al., 1970; Whitehead et al., 1975; Cheli and Aste, 1976) has undoubtedly contributed to the current confusion regarding duodenitis and its relationship to duodenal ulcer. To a large extent this has been due to a failure to appreciate the range of normal appearances in biopsies from the duodenal bulb (Kreuning, 1978). The diagnosis of duodenitis will be considered with respect to changes affecting villous architecture, inflammatory cell infiltrate, surface and crypt epithelium, and Brunner's glands.

(a) *Villous architecture.* There is considerable variation in shape and length of villi in the normal duodenal bulb with leaf-shaped and clubbed forms being common, and suitably orientated sections of biopsies will reflect this (Section 10.2.1). In a superficial biopsy, not including the muscularis mucosae, blunting and broadening of the villi may be accentuated, and focal effacement of the villous architecture may occur associated with lymphoid follicles or intramucosal lobules of Brunner's glands. Because of this, apparent alterations in villous architecture have to be interpreted with caution and not assessed in isolation.

(b) *Inflammatory cell infiltrate.* The content of lymphocytes and plasma cells in the normal mucosa of the first part of the duodenum varies and this may be apparent even within a single biopsy (Kreuning, 1978). For this reason the diagnosis and grading of duodenitis on this criterion alone is unreliable. The most valuable indicator of inflammation, which appears to correlate best with a visually abnormal bulb at endoscopy (Cotton et al., 1973; McCallum et al., 1979; Hasan et al., 1981), is the presence of neutrophil polymorphs in the lamina propria and infiltrating the epithelium of the crypts and surface epithelium (Figs 11.1 and 11.2). This

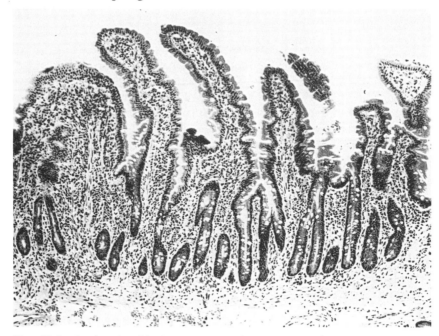

Fig. 11.1 A questionable increase in inflammatory cells is present in this duodenal bulb biopsy. HE × 93.

change is often focal and may be restricted to one part of the biopsy. It is important therefore to examine different levels and, where duodenitis is suspected at endoscopy or clinically, multiple biopsies should be taken. When there is a heavy plasma cell and lymphocytic infiltrate in the mucosa a careful search will almost invariably reveal some acute inflammatory cells as well. Other features of active inflammation such as vascular dilatation and oedema are occasionally a prominent feature (Fig. 11.3). Increasing degrees of mucosal inflammation are associated with progressive villous obliteration (Fig. 11.4) which in its severest form results in a flat mucosa.

(c) *Surface and crypt epithelium.* Associated with active mucosal inflammation are reactive and degenerative changes of the surface epithelium with increased basophilia of the cytoplasm, reduction in cell height and nuclear hyperchromasia (Fig. 11.5). These changes are most marked and often restricted to the villous epithelium although in severe inflammation crypt epithelium may also be affected. Regenerative changes may take the form of syncytial masses of epithelial cells projecting from the surface. When active inflammation is severe foci of superficial erosion may occur (Fig. 11.6).

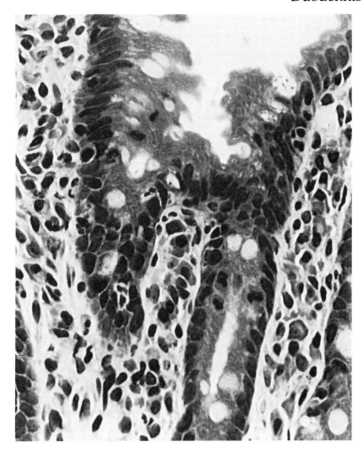

Fig. 11.2 Higher power of Fig. 11.1 shows scattered neutrophils in the lamina propria and epithelium. HE × 600.

A common change in duodenitis is so-called gastric metaplasia where groups of mucin-secreting cells identical to those of the gastric mucosa develop in the surface epithelium (James, 1964). A section stained with the PAS technique is helpful in delineating these cells (Fig. 11.7). It is not clear whether they originate from Brunner's glands or from undifferentiated crypt cells. Gastric metaplasia has been experimentally induced following excessive exposure to acid (Florey *et al.*, 1939; Rhodes, 1964) and it is a common feature in duodenal ulcer patients with high acid levels (Patrick *et al.*, 1974) suggesting that it develops as a protective mechanism. However the extent of the change does not correlate with peak acid output (Patrick *et al.*, 1974; Kreuning, 1978) and it may occur in hypochlorhydric individuals and in other inflammatory conditions such

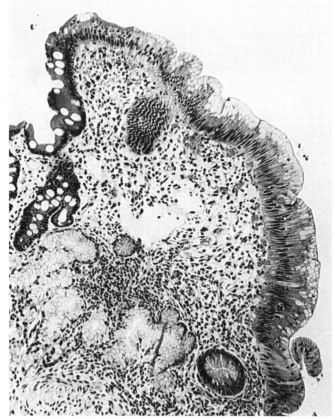

Fig. 11.3   Active duodenitis. Oedema of the lamina propria and polymorphs in surface epithelium. Prominent gastric metaplasia. HE × 135.

as Crohn's disease. As well as this it can be an isolated change unassociated with duodenal inflammation, when it is the tips of the villi which are affected (Fig. 10.3). In a recent study this focal superficial gastric metaplasia was seen in a majority of duodenal bulb biopsies from healthy volunteers (Kreuning *et al.*, 1978).

(d) *Brunner's glands.* Hyperplasia of Brunner's glands, sometimes resulting in nodularity of the mucosa of the duodenal bulb, has been described in association with duodenitis (Maratka *et al.*, 1979; Franzin *et al.*, 1982). It has been suggested that this change is a response to hypersecretion of acid but no such obvious correlation exists (Stokes *et al.*, 1964; Patrick *et al.*, 1974). It has been proposed that the diagnosis can be made by finding lobulated Brunner's glands in the mucosa above a fenestrated muscularis mucosae (Maratka *et al.*, 1979). However in the study of Kreuning *et al.* (1978) this occurred in the duodenal bulb biopsies of 48 out of 50 healthy volunteers, so that assessment would appear unsatisfactory in biopsy material. Extension of inflammatory cells between Brunner's glands may be present in some cases of duodenitis.

11.1.3   Summary

The significance of duodenitis and its relationship to duodenal ulceration continues to be debated. The reasons for this include the differing clinical, endoscopic and histological criteria used to make the diagnosis, the variability of symptoms experienced by patients with 'duodenitis' and the usually patchy nature of the inflammation. Because of the latter it is important that multiple adequate sized biopsies are taken from the duodenal bulb when the diagnosis is suspected clinically. The presence of acute inflammatory cells in biopsy material appears to correlate best with symptoms of non-ulcer dyspepsia (Cotton *et al.*, 1973; Joffe *et al.*, 1978) and a subjective grading into minor, moderate or severe degrees of active inflammation may be made on the basis of their prevalence.

Although in a few instances the progression from duodenitis to

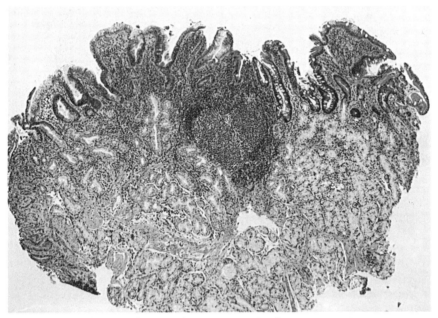

Fig. 11.4   Duodenitis. There is a heavy mucosal inflammatory cell infiltrate with widening and blunting of villi. HE × 55.

duodenal ulcer has been clearly documented (Cotton *et al.*, 1973; Thomson *et al.*, 1977) and the type of inflammation (Hasan *et al.*, 1983), its distribution (Paoluzi *et al.*, 1982) and the pattern of mucosal cell proliferation (Bransom *et al.*, 1981) is similar in the two conditions, further careful clinical and histopathological follow-up studies are needed to determine the natural history of chronic non-specific duodenitis.

11.2   Coeliac disease

Several studies have shown that biopsies from the second part of the duodenum at upper gastrointestinal endoscopy are as satisfactory as

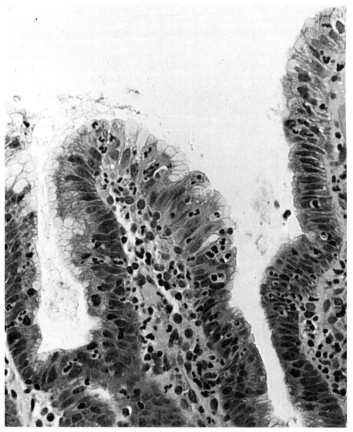

Fig. 11.5   Duodenitis. Higher power of Fig. 11.4 shows numerous polymorphs, regenerative changes in epithelium and gastric metaplasia. HE × 375.

Fig. 11.6   Duodenitis. Erosion with fibrinopurulent exudate. HE × 132.
Fig. 11.7   Gastric metaplasia affecting several villi. PAS/AB × 150.

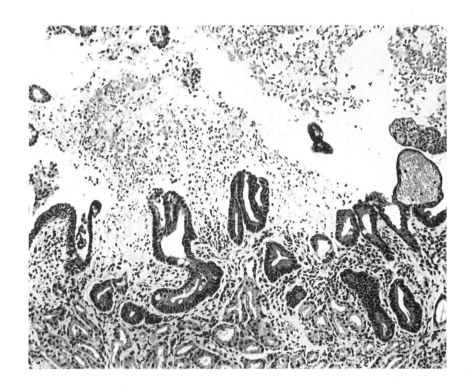

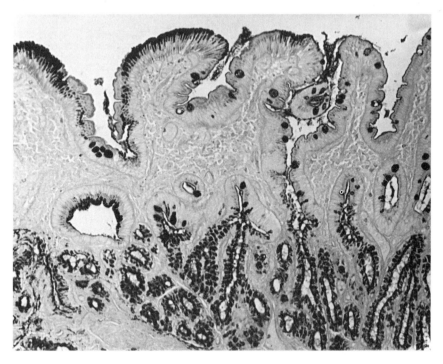

standard capsule methods in diagnosing coeliac disease (Stevens and McCarthy 1976; Holdstock *et al.*, 1979; Scott and Jenkins, 1981) and indeed offer some advantages. These include observation of the small intestine with the opportunity to take directed biopsies together with the option of dye scattering techniques to facilitate assessment of villous morphology (Stevens and McCarthy, 1976). As well as this the mucosa of the oesophagus and stomach can be examined at the same time.

Because of patchiness of the mucosal abnormality (Scott and Losowsky, 1976) several biopsies should be taken and these should ideally be orientated mucosal surface upwards on plastic mesh or a ground glass slide with the aid of a dissecting microscope, and placed immediately in fixative. The size of the samples are comparable to those obtained via a capsule if endoscopes with a large biopsy channel are used (Fig. 1.2).

Biopsies taken only from the first part of the duodenum are not entirely satisfactory for two reasons. Firstly, as mentioned previously, some degree of broadening and blunting of villi is normal for this part of the duodenum, and secondly, difficulty may arise in differentiating the changes from those seen in non-specific chronic (peptic) duodenitis, which primarily affects the duodenal bulb. If changes suggesting the latter are present endoscopically in a patient in whom coeliac disease is suspected then multiple biopsies from both the first and second parts of the duodenum should be taken. This will usually enable differentiation to be made between duodenitis occurring alone and duodenitis in conjunction with coeliac disease, when it may be a factor preventing a complete response to gluten withdrawal (Bayless *et al.*, 1982).

Detailed consideration of the histological appearances of coeliac disease will not be considered here but merely an outline of those features which help to distinguish it from non-specific duodenitis.

In untreated coeliac disease the mucosa is flat (Fig. 11.8) or shows shortened and thickened villi. There is a marked increase in plasma cells in the lamina propria which often have a tendency to predominate in the upper half of the mucosa. The total number of lymphocytes is not raised but their distribution alters, with large numbers infiltrating between epithelial cells. Eosinophils may also be conspicuous in the lamina propria but polymorphs are usually absent or limited in number. Surface enterocytes are distorted and crowded together (Fig. 11.9). Commensurate architectural changes are unusual in non-specific duodenitis and when present are associated with considerable active inflammation with polymorphs in the lamina propria and often infiltrating crypt and surface epithelium. Regenerative epithelial changes are present in association with this but the nuclear crowding and interepithelial lymphocytes characteristic of coeliac disease are not seen in non-inflamed areas of the

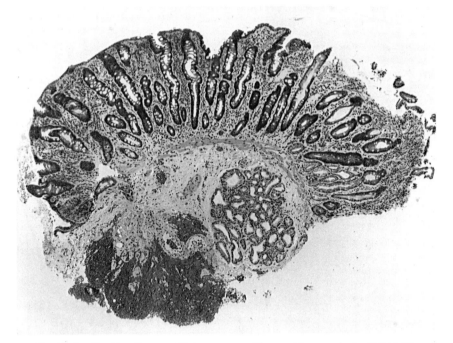

Fig. 11.8   Coeliac disease. Flat mucosa with crypt hyperplasia. HE × 50.

surface epithelium. In the majority of cases the distinction between the two conditions is straightforward particularly when clinical and endoscopic findings and the distribution of the changes in the duodenum are taken into account.

11.3   Crohn's disease

Symptomatic involvement of the duodenum, with or without concomitant gastric involvement, is uncommon in Crohn's disease and occurred in 4 and 2.2% of patients respectively in two large series (Fielding *et al.*, 1970; Rutgeerts *et al.*, 1980). In most cases it coincides with or follows lower intestinal disease but occasionally it antedates disease elsewhere or is confined to the upper gastrointestinal tract (Nugent *et al.*, 1977). Symptoms may be similar to those of a peptic ulcer, which indeed is not an uncommon accompaniment of Crohn's disease (Fielding and Cooke, 1970). Epigastric pain is rarely severe however and nausea and vomiting, often with temporary relief of symptoms, are common. There can be haemetemesis or melaena and weight loss is frequent.

Appearances at endoscopy are variable and include thickening of the mucosal folds, sometimes associated with focal nodularity, diffuse

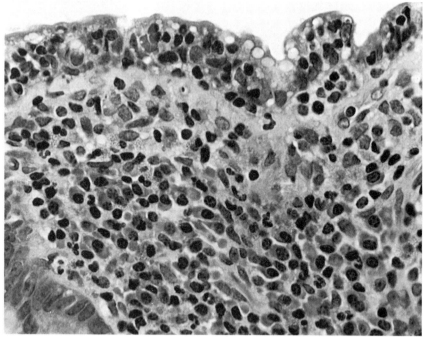

Fig. 11.9 Coeliac disease. Numerous lymphocytes are present in the surface epithelium which consists of crowded enterocytes with a multi-layered appearance. Note increased cellularity of the lamina propria in which plasma cells are conspicuous. HE × 600.

nodularity and fissuring ulceration giving a cobblestone appearance, and ulcers and erosions, which are usually multiple, aphthous-like or with a serpiginous outline and occur most frequently beyond the duodenal bulb. There can be lack of distensibility of the involved area, and endoscopic examination of the bulb may not be possible when stenotic disease affects the gastric outlet.

The changes in biopsies reflect the patchy nature of the inflammation and vary from normal mucosa to non-specific inflammation in which gastric and pyloric gland metaplasia may be present. Non-caseating epithelioid cell granulomas (Fig. 11.10) have been identified with varying success (Nugent *et al.*, 1977; Rutgeerts *et al.*, 1980). In surgical resection specimens from the upper gastrointestinal tract, granulomas are more common in the mucosa than in other layers (Haggitt and Meissner, 1973) and in a recent biopsy study were found incidentally in 7% of patients with proven Crohn's disease elsewhere but with no clinical, radiological or endoscopic evidence of duodenal involvement (Korelitz *et al.*, 1981).

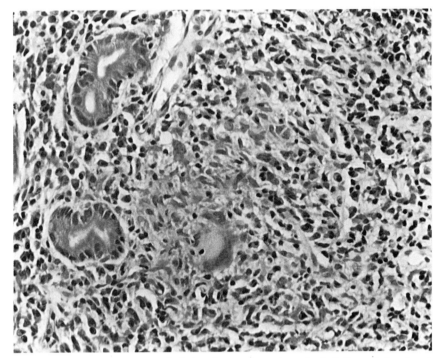

Fig. 11.10   Crohn's disease. Ill-defined granuloma in actively inflamed duodenal mucosa. HE × 360.

11.4   Giardiasis

The flagellate protozoon *Giardia lamblia* is the commonest intestinal parasite in many of the countries of Europe and in the USA. In a study from Norway, cysts were identified in the stools of 3.2% of an unselected hospital group (Petersen, 1972). The vegetative trophozoites reside in the duodenum and upper small intestine and encystment usually occurs in the lower ileum. There is no doubt that in a proportion of individuals infestation results in symptoms such as abdominal discomfort, flatulence, and diarrhoea, which may be acute, or chronic and intermittent. In the severest cases there can be steatorrhoea (Wright *et al.*, 1977). Many of these have occurred following travel abroad (Brodsky *et al.*, 1974) and epidemiological evidence points to contaminated water supplies as the vehicle of infection. Giardiasis may occur in coeliac disease (Carswell *et al.*, 1973), following partial gastrectomy (Yardley *et al.*, 1964), in alpha-chain disease (Section 12.5), and in gastrointestinal immunodeficiency syndromes (Ament and Rubin, 1972), notably in hypogammaglobulinaemia associated with nodular lymphoid hyperplasia of the small intestine (Hermans *et al.*, 1966). In some individuals with chronic Giardia infection and normal serum levels of immunoglobulins, low levels of secretory IgA have been present in duodenal aspirates (Zinneman and Kaplan, 1972). Defective cellular cytotoxity for Giardia (Smith *et al.*, 1982) and possession of particular HLA antigens (Roberts-Thomson *et al.*, 1980) have also been implicated in prolonged infections.

In biopsies of the duodenum and jejunum, trophozoites are most numerous in the zone between the crypts and the tips of the villi (Figs 11.11 and 11.12) and mostly appear as sickle-shaped bodies with their concave surface facing the epithelium. Less commonly they are sectioned coronally when they are pear-shaped, bilaterally symmetrical, from 10–21 µm long and 5–15 µm wide and with two large nuclei anteriorly. They are readily apparent in sections stained with haematoxylin and eosin and

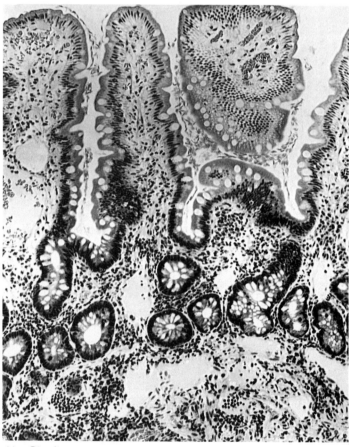

Fig. 11.11   Giardiasis. Numerous protozoa apposed to sides of villi. HE × 150.

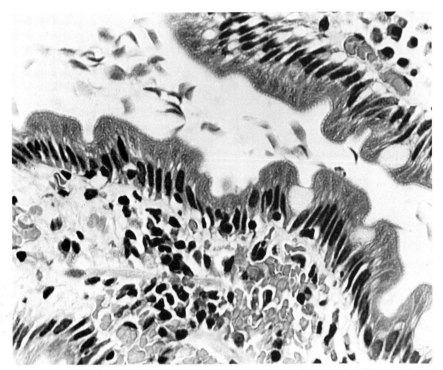

Fig. 11.12   Giardiasis. Some organisms sectioned coronally. HE × 600.

may also be demonstrated in Giemsa-stained impression smears or in duodenal aspirates. In one report a differential staining technique (Brandborg *et al.*, 1967) demonstrated organisms in the epithelium, lamina propria and submucosa of the small intestine and they have also been observed at an ultrastructural level within the mucosa (Morecki and Parker, 1967).

Although the mucosa usually appears normal even when numerous organisms are present, varying degrees of villous atrophy have been described which have reverted to normal following specific treatment of the infection (Alp and Hislop, 1969; Wright *et al.*, 1977; Levinson and Nastro, 1978). These have all been in symptomatic individuals many of whom have had malabsorption. Five of six patients studied by Yardley *et al.* (1964) with giardiasis and malabsorption showed focal acute inflammation of the crypts in jejunal biopsies. More often however the mucosa has appeared normal even when malabsorption has been present.

In cases of nodular lymphoid hyperplasia with hypogammaglobulinaemia a characteristic endoscopic appearance is present in the duodenum with numerous smooth surfaced hemispherical nodules from one to a few millimetres in diameter. Histologically, enlarged lymphoid follicles within the lamina propria are seen (Fig. 11.13) with effacement of the villous pattern overlying them but which is normal elsewhere. The follicles have prominent germinal centres with clear-cut margins. Plasma cells are inconspicuous or absent in the mucosa and trophozoites of Giardia are almost invariably present in relation to the epithelium of the surface and crypts.

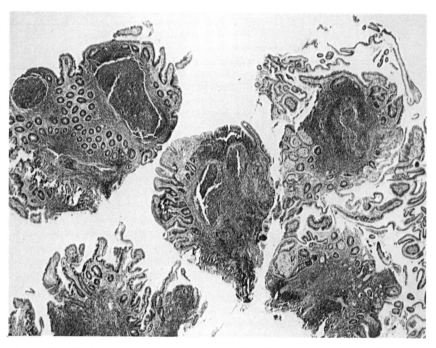

Fig. 11.13   Nodular lymphoid hyperplasia. Giardia present but not visible at this magnification. Biopsies from patient with hypogammaglobulinaemia. HE × 28.5.

11.5   Other causes of duodenitis

Inflammation of the descending duodenum with enlargement, hyperaemia and friability of mucosal folds in the region of the papilla can occur in acute or chronic pancreatitis (Blackstone and Mizuno, 1977; Makrauer *et al.*, 1982), and an erosive gastroduodenitis has been described secondary to chronic abdominal vascular insufficiency (Allende and Ona, 1982).

Various parasitic infestations which may be obscure causes of duodenitis in non-endemic areas have been diagnosed following upper endoscopy and biopsy. They include schistosomiasis due to *Schistosoma mansoni* (Witham and Mosser, 1979) and strongyloidiasis. Bone *et al.*, (1982) described a case of the latter in which florid hypertrophy and inflammation resulted in virtual occlusion of the lumen of the second part of the duodenum.

Tuberculous infection of the small intestine is usually a late complication of pulmonary disease, but very rarely primary disease may present with duodenal involvement (Lockwood *et al.*, 1974).

References

Allende, H. D. and Ona, F. V. (1982), Celiac artery and superior mesenteric artery insufficiency. Unusual cause of erosive gastroduodenitis. *Gastroenterology*, **82**, 763–766.

Alp, M. H. and Hislop, I. G. (1969), The effect of *Giardia lamblia* infestation on the gastrointestinal tract. *Aust. Ann. Med.*, **18**, 232–237.

Ament, M. E. and Rubin, C. E. (1972), Relation of giardiasis to abnormal intestinal structure and function in gastrointestinal immunodeficiency syndromes. *Gastroenterology*, **62**, 216–226.

Aronson, A. R. and Norfleet, R. G. (1962), The duodenal mucosa in peptic ulcer disease. A clinical pathological correlation. *Am. J. Dig. Dis.*, **7**, 506–514.

Bayless, T. M., Jones, B., Hamilton, S. R. and Yardley, J. H. (1982), Nodular duodenal bulb and peptic duodenitis in incompletely responsive 'atypical' sprue. *Gastroenterology*, **82**, 1014 (abstract).

Beck, I. T., Kahn, D. S., Lacerte, M. *et al.* (1965), 'Chronic duodenitis': a clinical pathological entity? *Gut*, **6**, 376–383.

Blackstone, M. O. and Mizuno, H. (1977), Reactive duodenal changes in chronic pancreatitis simulating the contiguous spread of pancreatic carcinoma. *Dig. Dis.*, **22**, 658–661.

Bone, M. F., Chesner, I. M., Oliver, R. and Asquith, P. (1982), Endoscopic appearances of duodenitis due to strongyloidiasis. *Gastrointest. Endosc.*, **28**, 190–191.

Brandborg, L. L., Tankersley, C. B., Gottlieb, S. *et al.* (1967), Histological demonstration of mucosal invasion by *Giardia lamblia* in man. *Gastroenterology*, **52**, 143–150.

Bransom, C. J., Boxer, M. E., Palmar, K. R. *et al.* (1981), Mucosal cell proliferation in duodenal ulcer and duodenitis. *Gut*, **22**, 277–282.

Brodsky, R. E., Spencer, H. C. and Schultz, M. G. (1974), Giardiasis in American travellers to the Soviet Union. *J. Infect. Dis.*, **130**, 319–323.

Carswell, F., Gibson, A. A. M. and McAllister, T. A. (1973), Giardiasis and coeliac disease. *Arch. Dis. Child.*, **48**, 414–418.

Cheli, R. and Aste, H. (1976), *Duodenitis*, Georg Thieme, Stuttgart, pp. 63–64.

Classen, M., Koch, H. and Demling, L. (1970), Duodenitis. Significance and frequency. *Bibl. Gastroenterol.*, **9**, 48–69.

Cotton, P. B., Price, A. B., Tighe, J. R. and Beales, J. S. M. (1973), Preliminary evaluation of 'duodenitis' by endoscopy and biopsy. *Br. Med. J.*, **3**, 430–433.

Fielding, J. F. and Cooke, W. T. (1970), Peptic ulceration in Crohn's disease (regional enteritis). *Gut*, **11**, 998–1000.

Fielding, J. F., Toye, D. K. M., Beton, D. C. and Cooke, W. T. (1970), Crohn's disease of the stomach and duodenum. *Gut*, **11**, 1001–1006.

Florey, H. W., Jennings, M. A., Jennings, D. A. and O'Connor, R. C. (1939), The reactions of the intestine of the pig to gastric juice. *J. Pathol. Bact.*, **49**, 105–123.

Franzin, G., Musola, R. and Mencarelli, R. (1982), Changes in the mucosa of the stomach and duodenum during immunosuppressive therapy after renal transplantation. *Histopathology*, **6**, 439–449.

Gelzayd, E. A., Gelfand, D. W. and Rinaldo, J. A. Jr. (1973), Non-specific duodenitis: a distinct clinical entity? *Gastrointest. Endosc.*, **19**, 131–133.

Gregg, J. A. and Garabedian, M. (1974), Duodenitis. *Am. J. Gastroenterol.*, **61**, 177–184.

Haggitt, R. C. and Meissner, W. A. (1973), Crohn's disease of the upper gastrointestinal tract. *Am. J. Clin. Pathol.*, **59**, 613–622.

Hasan, M., Sircus, W. and Ferguson, A. (1981), Duodenal mucosal architecture in non-specific and ulcer-associated duodenitis. *Gut*, **22**, 637–641.

Hasan, M., Hay, F., Sircus, W. and Ferguson, A. (1983), Nature of the inflammatory cell infiltrate in duodenitis. *J. Clin. Pathol.*, **36**, 280–288.

Hermans, P. E., Huizenga, K. A., Hoffman, H. N. II. *et al.* (1966), Dysgammaglobulinemia associated with nodular lymphoid hyperplasia of the small intestine. *Am. J. Med.*, **40**, 78–89.

Holdstock, G., Eade, O. E., Isaacson, P. and Smith, C. L. (1979), Endoscopic duodenal biopsies in coeliac disease and duodenitis. *Scand. J. Gastroenterol.*, **14**, 717–720.

James, A. H. (1964), Gastric epithelium in the duodenum. *Gut*, **5**, 285–294.

Joffe, S. N., Lee, F. D. and Blumgart, L. H. (1978), Duodenitis. *Clin. Gastroenterol.*, **7**, 635–650.

Korelitz, B. I., Waye, J. D., Kreuning, J. *et al.* (1981), Crohn's disease in endoscopic biopsies of the gastric antrum and duodenum. *Am. J. Gastroenterol.*, **76**, 103–109.

Kreuning, J. (1978), *Chronic Non-specific Duodenitis. A Clinical and Histopathological Study.* W. D. Meinema, Delft.

Kreuning, J., Bosman, F. T., Kuiper, G. *et al.* (1978), Gastric and duodenal mucosa in 'healthy' individuals. An endoscopic and histopathological study of 50 volunteers. *J. Clin. Pathol.*, **31**, 69–77.

Levinson, J. D. and Nastro, L. J. (1978), Giardiasis with total villous atrophy. *Gastroenterology*, **74**, 271–275.

Lockwood, C. M., Forster, P. M., Forbes Catto, J. V. and Stewart, J. S. (1974), A case of duodenal tuberculosis. *Dig. Dis.*, **19**, 575–579.

McCallum, R. W., Singh, D. and Wollman, J. (1979), Endoscopic and histologic correlations of the duodenal bulb. The spectrum of duodenitis. *Arch. Pathol.*, **103**, 169–172.

Makrauer, F. L., Antonioli, D. A. and Banks, P. A. (1982), Duodenal stenosis in chronic pancreatitis. Clinicopathological correlations. *Dig. Dis. Sci.*, **27**, 525–532.

Maratka, Z., Kocianova, J., Kudrmann, J. *et al.* (1979), Hyperplasia of Brunner's glands. Radiology, endoscopy and biopsy findings in 11 cases of diffuse, nodular and adenomatous form. *Acta Hepato-Gastroenterol.*, **26**, 64–69.

Morecki, R. and Parker, J. G. (1967), Ultrastructural studies of the human *Giardia lamblia* and subjacent jejunal mucosa in a subject with steatorrhea. *Gastroenterology*, **52**, 151–164.

Nebel, O. T., Farrell, R. L., Kirchner, J. P. and Macionus, R. F. (1973), Duodenoscopy in the evaluation of patients with upper gastrointestinal symptoms. *Gastrointest. Endosc.*, **19**, 142–143.

Nugent, F. W., Richmond, M. and Park, S. K. (1977), Crohn's disease of the duodenum. *Gut*, **18**, 115–120.

Paoluzi, P., Pallone, F., Palazzesi, P. *et al.* (1982), Frequency and extent of bulbar duodenitis in duodenal ulcer, endoscopic and histological study. *Endoscopy*, **14**, 193–195.

Patrick, W. J. A., Denham, D. and Forrest, A. P. M. (1974), Mucous change in the human duodenum: a light and electron microscopic study and correlation with disease and gastric acid secretion. *Gut*, **15**, 767–776.

Petersen, H. (1972), Giardiasis (lambliasis). *Scand. J. Gastroenterol.*, **7**, 1–44 (suppl. 14).

Rhodes, J. (1964), Experimental production of gastric epithelium in the duodenum. *Gut*, **5**, 454–458.

Roberts-Thomson, I. C., Mitchell, G. F., Andres, R. F. *et al.* (1980), Genetic studies in human and murine giardiasis. *Gut*, **21**, 397–401.

Rutgeerts, P., Onette, E., Vantrappen, G. *et al.* (1980), Crohn's disease of the stomach and duodenum: a clinical study with emphasis on the value of endoscopy and endoscopic biopsies. *Endoscopy*, **12**, 288–294.

Scott, B. B. and Jenkins, D. (1981), Endoscopic small intestinal biopsy. *Gastrointest. Endosc.*, **27**, 162–167.

Scott, B. B. and Losowsky, M. S. (1976), Patchiness and duodenal-jejunal variation of the mucosal abnormality in coeliac disease and dermatitis herpetiformis. *Gut*, **17**, 984–992.

Smith, P. D., Gillin, F. D., Spira, W. M. and Nash, T. E. (1982), Chronic giardiasis: studies on drug sensitivity, toxin production, and host immune response. *Gastroenterology*, **83**, 797–803.

Stevens, F. M. and McCarthy, C. F. (1976), The endoscopic demonstration of coeliac disease. *Endoscopy*, **8**, 177–180.

Stokes, J. F., Turnberg, L. A. and Hawksley, J. C. (1964), Hyperplasia of Brunner's glands. *Gut*, **5**, 459–462.

Thomson, W. O., Joffe, S. N., Robertson, A. G. *et al.* (1977), Is duodenitis a dyspeptic myth? *Lancet*, **i**, 1197–1198.

Whitehead, R., Roca, M., Meikle, D. D. *et al.* (1975), The histological classification of duodenitis in fibreoptic biopsy specimens. *Digestion*, **13**, 129–136.

Witham, R. R. and Mosser, R. S. (1979), An unusual presentation of schistosomiasis duodenitis. *Gastroenterology*, **77**, 1316–1318.

Wright, S. G., Tomkins, A. M. and Ridley, D. S. (1977), Giardiasis: clinical and therapeutic aspects. *Gut*, **18**, 343–350.

Yardley, J. H., Takano, J. and Hendrix, T. R. (1964), Epithelial and other mucosal lesions of the jejunum in giardiasis. Jejunal biopsy studies. *Bull. Johns Hopkins Hosp.*, **115**, 389–406.

Zinneman, H. H. and Kaplan, A. P. (1972), The association of giardiasis with reduced intestinal secretory immunoglobulin A. *Dig. Dis.*, **17**, 793–797.

12 Non-neoplastic polyps and tumours of the duodenum

The duodenum is an uncommon site for neoplasms although endoscopy has shown that they are not as rare as autopsy studies would indicate. Thus in a recent series from a referral centre they were encountered in 1% of duodenoscopies (Wald and Milligan, 1975). Many of the tumours, particularly those arising from the mucosa, are polypoid and may be biopsied or removed whole. However, because of the small diameter of the lumen, polypectomy is technically difficult and even when accomplished it may be impossible to retrieve the polyp via the pylorus. Snare polypectomy with electrocoagulation in the second part of the duodenum has been followed by transient pancreatitis (Alper *et al.*, 1975).

Before discussing tumours of the duodenum non-neoplastic polyps at this site will be considered. They include hyperplasia of lymphoid tissue (Section 11.4), Brunner's gland hyperplasia, ectopic gastric and pancreatic tissue, and Peutz-Jegher's polyps. Rare cases of inflammatory fibroid polyps (Section 8.1.5) in this site have been recorded (Ott *et al.*, 1980).

12.1 Non-neoplastic polyps

12.1.1 Brunner's gland hyperplasia

Hyperplasia of Brunner's glands can result in discrete, circumscribed, sessile polyps predominantly affecting the first part of the duodenum, or be a diffuse process with involvement of more distal parts and a nodular or cobblestone appearance of the mucosa at endoscopy. There has been an inconstant association in reported cases with inflammation in the duodenum and with acid hypersecretion (Stokes *et al.*, 1964; de Castella, 1966; Maratka *et al.*, 1979). In a recent study Paimela *et al.* (1984) found it to be a common change in patients with chronic renal failure. In this group gastric acid secretion was normal, although there were significantly raised serum gastrin and pepsinogen I levels.

Endoscopic biopsies, because of their size and superficial nature, are not particularly helpful in diagnosis although they may serve to exclude other conditions such as nodular lymphoid hyperplasia, alpha-chain disease and involvement by Crohn's disease, which can give similar endoscopic appearances.

Rarely, single polyps occur which can reach several centimetres in diameter, when they are usually pedunculated. Although commonly referred to as 'adenomas' they are not true tumours and probably hyperplastic or hamartomatous. These larger lesions can bleed (Osborne *et al.*, 1973), obstruct the pylorus, or result in intussusception.

Microscopic examination shows numerous lobules of normal-appearing Brunner's glands divided by strands of smooth muscle from the muscularis mucosae (Fig. 12.1). Focal aggregates of lymphocytes can

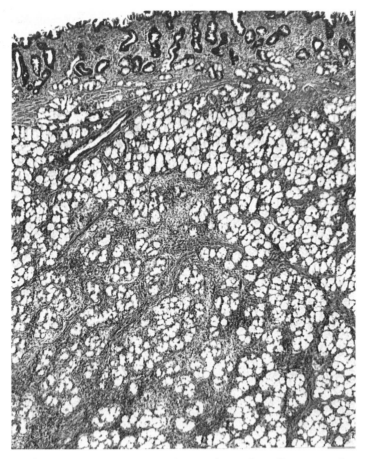

Fig. 12.1 Brunner's gland adenoma. Section from a 3 cm diameter pedunculated polyp in the duodenal bulb. HE × 37.

occur in the stroma, and cystic dilatation may be present, in some cases resulting in a mucocoele (Miyawaki and Straehley, 1973; Wolk *et al.*, 1973).

12.1.2   Ectopic gastric mucosa

Focal collections of orderly gastric glands consisting of chief and parietal cells and overlain by a surface epithelium of gastric type (Fig. 12.2) have been described in some 1 to 3% of endoscopies (Kreuning *et al.*, 1978; Lessells and Martin, 1982; Spiller *et al.*, 1982). At endoscopy the characteristic appearance is of multiple pink or red mucosal nodules usually under 1 cm in diameter mostly occurring on the anterior wall of the duodenal bulb. They are to be differentiated from metaplastic changes affecting the surface epithelium (Section 11.1.2(c)) and the presence of occasional parietal cells and less commonly chief cells which have been reported particularly in association with hypersecretion of acid and duodenal ulcer (Hoedemaeker, 1970; Franzin *et al.*, 1982). Their clinical significance is uncertain. There has been an inconstant association with gastric acid secretion (Johansen and Hart Hansen, 1973; Spiller *et al.*, 1982). It is possible they may be congenital.

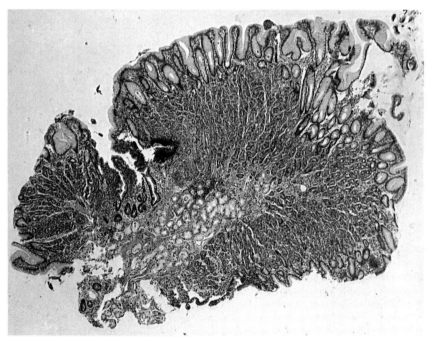

Fig. 12.2   Ectopic gastric mucosa. Note submucosal Brunner's glands. HE × 37.

12.1.3   Ectopic pancreatic tissue

Ectopic pancreatic tissue in the stomach and duodenum is a congenital abnormality thought to result from separation of fragments from the main mass of the pancreas during rotation of the foregut. At endoscopy the usual appearance of this uncommon lesion is indistinguishable from many other submucosal masses, namely a hemispherical sessile polyp, often with an umbilicated centre and of variable size, anything from a few millimetres to several centimetres in diameter. A distinctive feature of some has been the presence of an opening visible as a dimple on the surface. They are invariably single and the majority occur within 3 – 4 cm of either side of the pylorus (Zarling, 1981).

Histological examination shows pancreatic acini and ducts, in which cystic change is common, present in the submucosa (Fig. 12.3). Sectioning may disclose ducts leading to the lumen. Islets of Langerhans are present in approximately one-third of cases (Nickels and Laasonen, 1970). This pancreatic tissue may be accompanied by bundles of hypertrophied smooth muscle surrounding ducts lined by tall columnar or cuboidal epithelium along with collections of Brunner's glands, or the latter elements without pancreatic tissue may be found alone, where the term adenomyoma has been applied (Janota and Smith, 1966; Lasser and Koufman, 1977). Larger lesions near the pylorus produce symptoms of gastric outlet obstruction, and ulceration and bleeding may occur. Lesions near the ampulla can cause obstruction of the common bile duct (Bill *et al.*, 1982). The majority, however, are incidental findings.

12.1.4   Peutz-Jeghers polyps

Gastric and duodenal polyps occur in 40% of patients with the Peutz-Jeghers syndrome (Bartholomew *et al.*, 1962). They may be up to several centimetres in size but are usually pedunculated with a thin stalk and amenable therefore to snare polypectomy. Prophylactic removal of polyps at endoscopy has been advocated in the management of these cases (Williams *et al.*, 1982).

Histologically these hamartomatous polyps consist of a branching core of smooth muscle derived from the muscularis mucosae covered by cytologically normal epithelium with Paneth and endocrine cells normally sited at the base of the crypts (Figs 12.4 and 12.5). Focal areas of cystic change and ischaemic necrosis may be present.

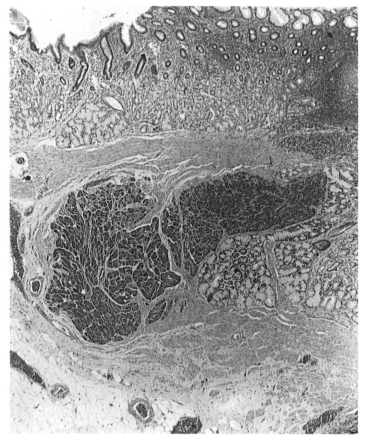

Fig. 12.3　Ectopic pancreas. Pancreatic acini and ducts in the submucosa of the stomach. HE × 36.

12.1.5　Other lesions

Lymphangiectatic cysts have been identified at necropsy in 20% of small bowels examined (Shilkin *et al.*, 1968) and may be seen at endoscopy as discrete creamy nodules a few mm in diameter which if biopsied discharge a white milky fluid (Gangl *et al.*, 1980). Uni- or multilocular thin-walled cysts are present in the submucosa and occasionally extend into the mucosa. They are clinically insignificant and probably acquired lesions and have to be distinguished from intestinal lymphangiectasia, a generalized disorder occurring in children and young adults and associated with hypoproteinaemia, oedema and diarrhoea, often with steatorrhoea (Pomerantz and Waldmann, 1963). Biopsy appearances can be similar but endoscopic and clinical findings clearly differentiate the two.

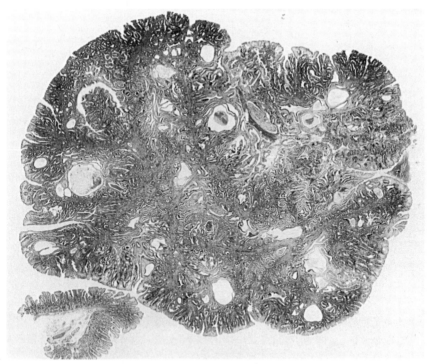

Fig. 12.4 Peutz-Jeghers polyp. HE × 7.

Angiomatous lesions may be observed at endoscopy and can cause symptoms of obstruction, intussusception and haemorrhage (Ikeda *et al.*, 1980). Vascular malformations may be present elsewhere particularly in the skin (Taylor and Torrance, 1974). Biopsy is not usually indicated.

12.2 Epithelial tumours

12.2.1 *Adenomas*

Adenomas of the duodenum are uncommon and in surgical series have often been quite large and have had a villous architecture. They are usually single and have been preferentially located in the second part. Pathological examination of resected specimens has shown that some 30 to 40% have undergone malignant change (Schulten *et al.*, 1976). As with large bowel adenomas the likelihood of this increases with increasing size (Perzin and Bridge, 1981).

Sporadic case reports of adenomas and carcinomas of the duodenum and bile ducts in patients with familial adenomatosis coli (Duncan *et al.*,

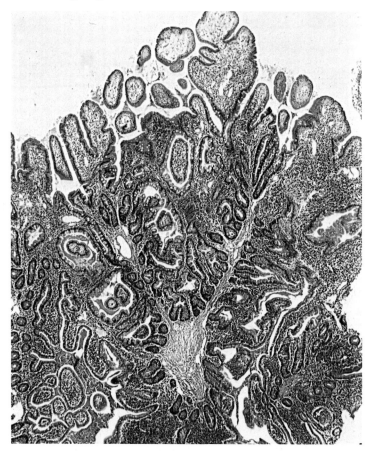

Fig. 12.5   Peutz-Jeghers polyp. Tree-like branching of the muscularis mucosae. HE × 37.

1968; Melmed and Bouchier, 1972) have indicated that neoplastic change is not confined to the large bowel, and recent endoscopic series have confirmed this in a high proportion of these individuals (Yao *et al.*, 1977; Ranzi *et al.*, 1981; Järvinen *et al.*, 1983). Single or more often multiple adenomas have been found in all parts of the duodenum although again most commonly in the second part particularly near the papilla (Fig. 12.6). Other duodenal polyps found in these patients have been non-neoplastic with cystic change affecting the epithelial crypts (Järvinen *et al.*, 1983), and analogous to the fundic glandular cysts in the stomach (Section 8.1.4(b)).

Histologically, adenomas consist of crowded, closely packed cells with hyperchromatic nuclei and numerous mitoses (Fig. 12.7). The cytological

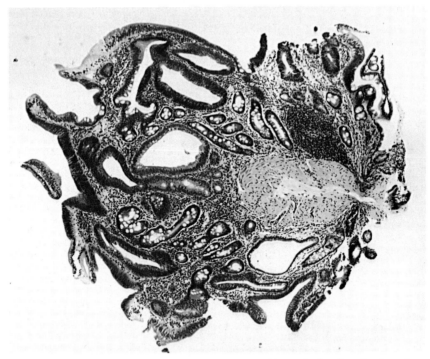

Fig. 12.6   Adenoma. Biopsy of one of several small sessile duodenal polyps in a patient with familial adenomatosis coli. HE × 60.

appearances are similar to adenomas of the stomach and large bowel and varying degrees of atypia can be present. In better differentiated tumours, absorptive, columnar, goblet, endocrine and Paneth cells may be identified (Mingazzini *et al.*, 1982). Multiple biopsies of these lesions are indicated for diagnosis and assessment of malignant change although sampling and the superficial nature of the material may preclude an accurate interpretation of the latter. Benign lesions may be removed locally at operation whereas more radical procedures are usually necess-ary for malignant tumours. Endoscopic removal of adenomas has also been achieved (Alper *et al.*, 1975; Dupas *et al.*, 1977).

12.2.2   Adenocarcinoma

Considering its length the duodenum is the favoured site in the small intestine for this tumour accounting for one third to one half of the total, although comprising only about 0.3% of all malignant gastrointestinal neoplasms. The majority of tumours are periampullary and with large

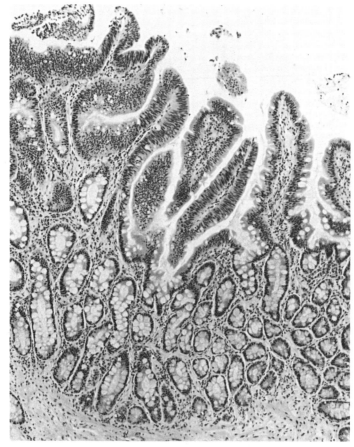

Fig. 12.7 Adenoma. Junction between villous adenoma showing moderate epithelial dysplasia and normal small intestinal mucosa. HE × 93.

lesions in this area distinction between primary tumours of the duodenal mucosa, papilla of Vater, bile ducts and pancreas may not be possible endoscopically or after histological examination of biopsies (Fig. 12.8). There is good evidence that the majority of duodenal adenocarcinomas arise from a pre-existing adenoma (Perzin and Bridge, 1981) and a villous component may be present in biopsy material (Fig. 12.9). As well as its

Fig. 12.8 Adenocarcinoma infiltrates the submucosa in this biopsy from the second part of the duodenum. Subsequently it was shown to arise from the head of the pancreas. HE × 60.

Fig. 12.9 Granulation tissue infiltrated by adenocarcinoma and separate fragment with villous structure. HE × 50.

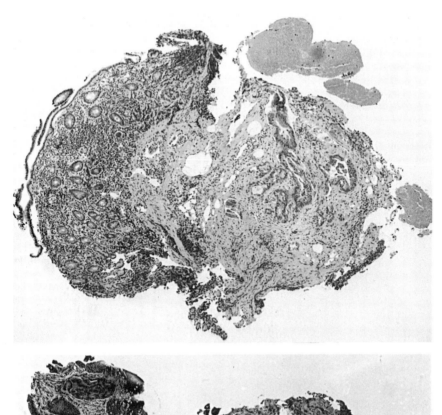

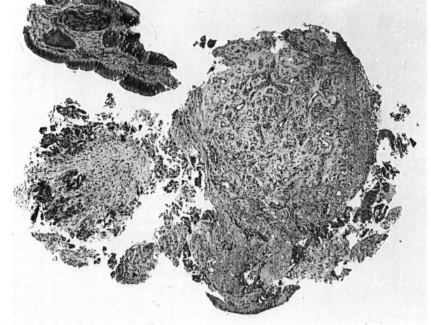

association with patients having familial adenomatosis coli (see above), adenocarcinoma of the upper small intestine is more common in people with coeliac disease than in the general population (Holmes *et al.*, 1980; Swinson *et al.*, 1983).

12.3   Endocrine cell tumours

It has been estimated that some 1 to 2.3% of endocrine cell tumours of the gastrointestinal tract occur in the duodenum (Martin and Potet, 1974), mostly in the first part. Macroscopically they may be polypoid, with an intact or eroded mucosa, or ulcerated, and are usually under 2 cm in diameter (Wilander *et al.*, 1979). The majority have not been associated with endocrine symptoms although radioimmunoassay and immuno-histochemical techniques have identified a large number of tumour products (often multiple in the same tumour) including gastrin, sub-stance P, VIP, (Figs 12.10, 12.11 and 12.12), glucagon, somatostatin, serotonin and catecholamines (Kaneko *et al.*, 1979; Roggli *et al.*, 1979;

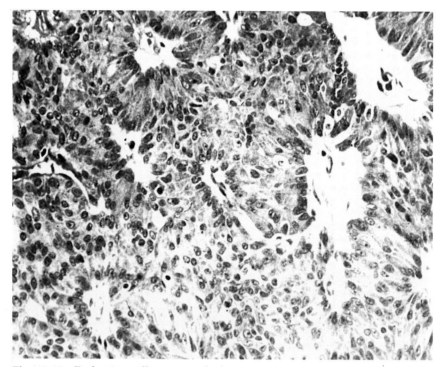

Fig. 12.10   Endocrine cell tumour which arose in the pancreas and invaded the duodenum. HE × 350.

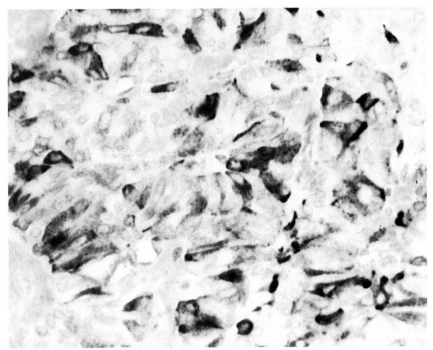

Fig. 12.11 Pancreatic Vipoma demonstrating pancreatic polypeptide-like immunoreactivity in many of the tumour cells. PAP × 450.

Wilander *et al.*, 1979). Duodenal gastrinomas, either alone or associated with pancreatic tumours, were present in 13% of 800 patients with the Zollinger-Ellison syndrome (Hofmann *et al.*, 1973).

Histologically, the tumours are characteristic of foregut carcinoids with a trabecular or ribbon pattern, although more solid or tubular areas can also be present. Mostly the tumours are argyrophilic with the Grimelius technique or Hellman-Hellestrom reaction and can also contain a few argentaffin cells (Wilander *et al.*, 1979). A distinctive group has recently been described (Griffiths *et al.*, 1983) with a small glandular pattern often associated with laminated calcified basophilic structures resembling psammoma bodies (Fig. 12.13). Immunohistochemical staining has demonstrated somatostatin in the tumour cells (Fig. 12.14). The tumours tend to be periampullary and some cases have occurred in patients with von Recklinghausen's disease and/or phaeochromocytoma (Hough *et al.*, 1983; Griffiths *et al.*, 1983). It has been suggested that this association may constitute a specific type of multiple endocrine neoplasia syndrome.

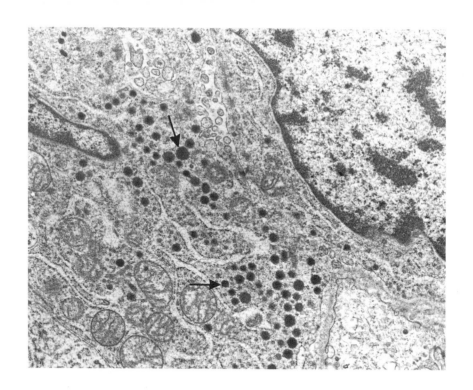

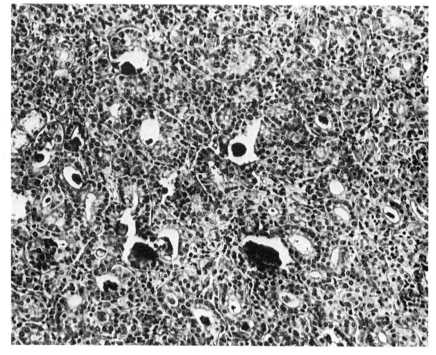

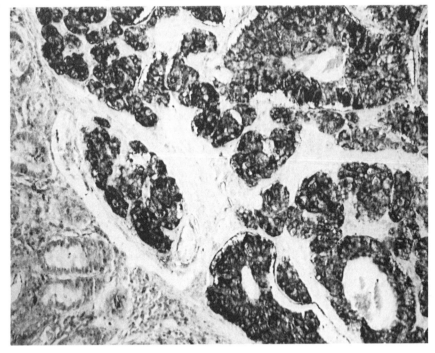

Fig. 12.14 Duodenal carcinoid tumour. Immunolocalization with anti-somatostatin. DNP hapten sandwich technique × 175.·

12.4   Connective tissue tumours

These include smooth muscle tumours, tumours derived from neural tissue, and lipomas. When benign these tumours only rarely cause symptoms, usually bleeding or obstruction, and are mostly incidental findings. Endoscopically they are seen as smooth hemispherical indentations overlain by a tense mucosa which is usually intact. Biopsies are usually non-contributory because they sample the overlying mucosa. Occasionally these tumours are polypoid and can be removed with the diathermy snare. Lipomas may be recognized by their soft consistency. A rare but distinctive duodenal tumour which occurs in the periampullary region is the so-called gangliocytic paraganglioma (Kepes and Zacharias, 1971). The majority of examples have been circumscribed, polypoid

Fig. 12.12   Electron photomicrograph showing secretory granules (arrowed) in a pancreatic Vipoma. × 18 000.

Fig. 12.13   Duodenal carcinoid with microglandular pattern. Note psammoma bodies. HE × 140.

lesions under 2 cm in diameter occurring in men (Taylor and Helwig, 1962). Invariably benign, on histological examination they are composed of clusters and ribbons of columnar epithelioid cells resembling the appearance seen in a chemodectoma, together with a usually less conspicuous spindle-cell component consisting of cells morphologically identical to Schwann cells. Some of the epithelioid cells, with more abundant cytoplasm and large round nuclei with prominent nucleoli, resemble ganglion cells.

Leiomyosarcomas, the commonest malignant mesenchymal tumour of the duodenum, comprise approximately 10% of malignant tumours at this site (Ochsner and Kleckner, 1957). The favoured areas are the second and third parts, emphasizing the importance of a thorough examination of the duodenum beyond the bulb in patients with undiagnosed gastro-intestinal haemorrhage. At the time of diagnosis these tumours are often large, and sinus or fistula formation may be demonstrated radiologically (Olurin and Solanke, 1968). As with smooth muscle tumours elsewhere in the gastrointestinal tract (see Section 9.5) the diagnosis of malignancy is often difficult to establish histologically and management may have to be based on endoscopic and clinical criteria (Yassinger *et al.*, 1977).

12.5   Malignant lymphomas

Primary lymphomas of the small bowel are almost as common as carcinomas but, unlike the latter, are preferentially located distally. The exceptions to this general statement are those lymphomas associated with malabsorptive states which tend to occur in the proximal parts of the small intestine. They can be divided into two groups. In countries of Western Europe and in the USA lymphomas have occurred in adults with known or presumptive coeliac disease (gluten-induced enteropathy). In the countries around the Mediterranean and in the Middle East lymphomas have affected children and young adults (so-called Mediterranean lymphomas) and have arisen on the basis of a diffuse proliferation of the gut-associated B lymphoid cells of the small intestine (immunoproliferative small intestinal disease – IPSID). In most instances this has been accompanied by the presence in the sera and secretions of immunoglobulin fragments, representing incomplete IgA heavy chains (alpha-chain disease).

Lymphomas occurring in adults with coeliac disease have been associated with a deterioration in the clinical picture with features such as diarrhoea, weight loss, abdominal pain, fever and occasionally finger clubbing (Freeman *et al.*, 1977). This may be followed by signs of peritonitis, associated with the perforation of one or more tumours, or of intestinal obstruction. In another group of patients, it is only after examination of the bowel following operation or necropsy and the finding of one or more ulcers or strictures with an intervening flat mucosa that allows a presumptive diagnosis of lymphoma complicating coeliac disease to be made. Histological study has shown an appearance varying from well differentiated histiocytes with only minimal atypia to sheets of monomorphic immature cells resembling poorly differentiated lymphoid malignancy or a highly pleomorphic tumour in which numerous multi-nucleated giant cells are present (Isaacson and Wright, 1980). Isaacson and Wright (1978) using immunological techniques have demonstrated, in individual tumour cells, the presence of both kappa and lambda light chains and all major classes of heavy chain, as well as lysozyme and alpha-1-antitrypsin, suggesting that the cells are phagocytic rather than lymphoid in origin; hence the name malignant histiocytosis. Multiple sections sometimes have to be examined before tumour cells are identified which has led to the suggestion that the 'benign' ulcers (non-granulomatous ulcerative jejuno-ileitis) described by others as a serious complication of coeliac disease (Bayless et al., 1967) probably represent a manifestation of malignant histiocytosis with secondary inflammation masking any malignant cells present. Whilst this is certainly so in some cases, ulceration unrelated to malignancy undoubtedly also occurs in the flat small intestinal mucosa (Robertson et al., 1983). There is no doubt also that some of these tumours are of follicle centre cell origin. They appear to be large cell diffuse lymphomas (centroblastic-Kiel classification) and the tumour cells have been negative for alpha-1-antichymotrypsin and lysozyme, although there are scattered macrophages of normal appearance within the tumour which do express these markers.

Because of the extremely poor prognosis of these tumours once perforation or haemorrhage has supervened, early changes which might indicate an increased risk of malignancy have been sought in resected material away from obviously malignant foci and retrospectively in biopsies from patients who subsequently developed tumours. Isaacson (1980) has described small collections of histiocytes with minimal or no atypia, frequently sited below the surface epithelium and sometimes invading it with resultant micro-erosion, or surrounding and destroying crypts (Fig. 12.15). These lesions have been focal and often only apparent when serial sections of biopsies have been examined. Others have observed an increase in the cellular infiltrate, particularly the content of plasma cells, which sometimes contain Russell bodies, together with eosinophils, occasional histiocytes and cells resembling reticulum cells (Whitehead, 1968).

The relationship of so-called coeliac disease in the adult to the child-hood form is another area which is not fully elucidated, in that the strict criteria employed for the diagnosis in children have seldom been applied

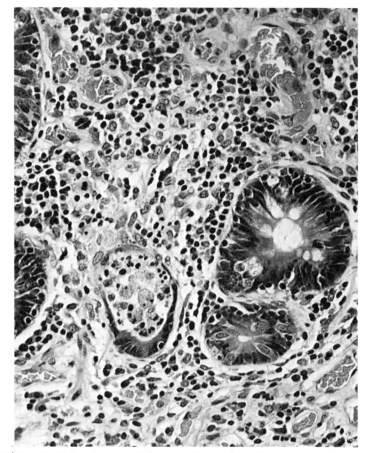

Fig. 12.15 Partially destroyed crypt with surrounding group of histiocytes. Possible early lesion indicating malignancy complicating coeliac disease. HE × 313.

to adults. Histological response to a gluten-free diet has been reported in adults (Freeman *et al.*, 1977) and the finding of similar HLA types as in childhood coeliac disease has also been documented (O'Driscoll *et al.*, 1982), so that available evidence is compatible with subclinical disease since childhood in adults presenting with malabsorption and with a flat small intestinal mucosa in whom other causes for this have been excluded. The significance of this relationship is that children with coeliac disease may also be at risk of developing malignant lymphomas of the small intestine and only long-term studies will determine the likelihood of this occurrence.

Immunoproliferative small intestinal disease (IPSID) occurs particularly in young people in the second and third decades who have a low socio-economic status and poor hygiene associated with a high frequency of acute infectious diarrhoeas and of parasitic infestations of the gut. Presentation is with a malabsorption syndrome resulting from extensive and diffuse infiltration of the wall of the small intestine predominantly by plasma cells. Immunoelectrophoresis of serum with monospecific antisera to IgA has detected alpha-chain protein in a majority of cases (Rambaud, 1983).

Three histological stages have been described in the small intestine (Galian *et al.*, 1977). In stage A the mucosa is thickened and the lamina propria expanded by a dense infiltrate of plasma cells, resulting in the enlargement and blunting of villi with crypt separation, although the surface epithelium usually remains remarkably unaffected (Fig. 12.16).

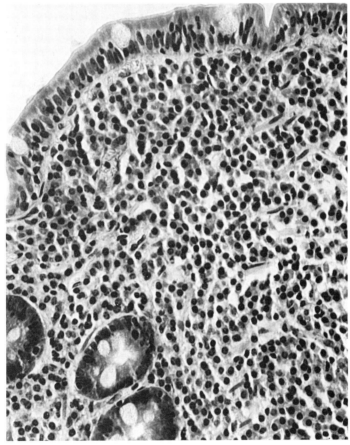

Fig. 12.16   Immunoproliferative small intestinal disease. Numerous plasma cells in the lamina propria. Note normal appearance of surface enterocytes. HE × 375.

There may be an increase in interepithelial lymphocytes. Trophozoites of *Giardia lamblia* are present in about one third of cases (Rambaud and Seligmann, 1976). In all cases associated with the detection of alpha-chain protein in the serum, and in a proportion of those where it is absent, immunoperoxidase studies show strong positive staining for IgA and J chain in nearly every cell but fail to stain with antisera to light chains (Asselah *et al.*, 1983). In stage C, lymphoma either extensively infiltrates the wall of the small bowel or forms circumscribed tumours, frequently sited in the jejunum. Stage B is a transitional phase, where pleomorphic lymphoplasmacytic cells (immunoblasts) are present in addition to plasma cells, and tend to infiltrate crypt epithelium and extend into the submucosa, sometimes aggregating to form small nodules. The lymphomas appear histologically to be of B cell type with plasma cell differentiation, although in general they fail to stain for any intracytoplasmic immunoglobulin class with the exception of faint staining for IgA and J chain in some of the cells of immunoblastic and lymphoplasmacytoid/lymphoplasmacytic lymphomas (Asselah *et al.*, 1983).

Direct inspection of the mucosa at duodenoscopy and jejunoscopy in cases of IPSID complicated by lymphoma has shown abnormalities in a high proportion of cases and enabled targeted biopsies to be taken (Barakat, 1982). The finding of definite evidence of malignancy in biopsies may make a staging or diagnostic laparotomy unnecessary. Although symptomatic relief has been obtained with antibiotics such as tetracycline and ampicillin, particularly in the early stages of the disease, relapse almost invariably occurs. Cytotoxic chemotherapy with or without steroids, and abdominal radiation have been used mostly in the later stages of the disease, but no results from controlled studies are available to assess their value in early disease compared with antibiotics alone.

References

Alper, E. I., Foroozan, P., Johnson, R. B. and Haubrich, W. S. (1975), Endoscopic polypectomy in the duodenum. Its complication by pancreatitis. *Gastrointest. Endosc.*, **21**, 119–122.

Asselah, F., Slavin, G., Sowter, G. and Asselah, H. (1983), Immunoproliferative small intestinal disease in Algerians. 1. Light microscopic and immunochemical studies. *Cancer*, **52**, 227–237.

Barakat, M. H. (1982), Endoscopic features of primary small bowel lymphoma: a proposed endoscopic classification. *Gut*, **23**, 36–41.

Bartholomew, L. G., Moore, C. E., Dahlin, D. C. and Waugh, J. M. (1962), Intestinal polyposis associated with mucocutaneous pigmentation. *Surg. Gynecol. Obstet.*, **115**, 1–11.

Bayless, T. M., Kapelowitz, R. F., Shelley, W. M. *et al.* (1967), Intestinal ulceration. A complication of celiac disease. *N. Engl. J. Med.*, **276**, 996–1002.

Bill, K., Belber, J. P. and Carson, J. W. (1982), Adenomyoma (pancreatic heterotopia) of the duodenum producing common bile duct obstruction. *Gastrointest. Endosc.*, **28**, 182–184.

de Castella, H. (1966), Brunner's gland adenoma. An unusual cause of intestinal bleeding. *Br. J. Surg.*, **53**, 153–156.

Duncan, B. R., Dohner, V. A. and Priest, J. H. (1968), The Gardner syndrome: need for early diagnosis. *J. Pediat.*, **72**, 497–505.

Dupas, J. L., Marti, R., Capron, J. P. and Delamarre, J. (1977), Villous adenoma of the duodenum. Endoscopic diagnosis and resection. *Endoscopy*, **9**, 245–247.

Franzin, G., Musola, R. and Mencarelli, R. (1982), Morphological changes of the gastroduodenal mucosa in regular dialysis uraemic patients. *Histopathology*, **6**, 429–437.

Freeman, H. J., Weinstein, W. M., Shnitka, T. K. *et al.* (1977), Primary abdominal lymphoma. Presenting manifestation of celiac sprue or complicating dermatitis herpetiformis. *Am. J. Med.*, **63**, 585–594.

Galian, A., Lecestre, M. J., Scotto, J. *et al.* (1977), Pathological studies of alpha-chain disease, with special emphasis on evolution. *Cancer*, **39**, 2081–2101.

Gangl, A., Polterauer, P., Krepler, R. and Kumpan, W. (1980), A further case of submucosal lymphangioma of the duodenum diagnosed during endoscopy. *Endoscopy*, **12**, 188–190.

Griffiths, D. F. R., Williams, G. T. and Williams, E. D. (1983), Multiple endocrine neoplasia associated with von Recklinghausen's disease. *Br. Med. J.*, **287**, 1341–1343.

Hoedemaeker, Ph.J. (1970), Heterotopic gastric mucosa in the duodenum. *Digestion*, **3**, 165–173.

Hofmann, J. W., Fox, P. S. and Wilson, S. D. (1973), Duodenal wall tumors and the Zollinger-Ellison syndrome. Surgical management. *Arch. Surg.*, **107**, 334–339.

Holmes, G. K. T., Dunn, G. I., Cockel, R. and Brookes, V. S. (1980), Adenocarcinoma of the upper small bowel complicating coeliac disease. *Gut*, **21**, 1010–1016.

Hough, D. R., Chan, A. and Davidson, H. (1983), Von Recklinghausen's disease associated with gastrointestinal carcinoid tumors. *Cancer*, **51**, 2206–2208.

Ikeda, K., Murayama, H., Takano, H. *et al.* (1980), Massive intestinal bleeding in hemangiomatosis of the duodenum. *Endoscopy*, **12**, 306–310.

Isaacson, P. (1980), Malignant histiocytosis of the intestine: the early histological lesion. *Gut*, **21**, 381–386.

Isaacson, P. and Wright, D. H. (1978), Malignant histiocytosis of the intestine: its relationship to malabsorption and ulcerative jejunitis. *Hum. Pathol.*, **9**, 661–677.

Isaacson, P. and Wright, D. H. (1980), Malabsorption and intestinal lymphomas. In *Recent Advances in Gastrointestinal Pathology* (ed. R. Wright), W. B. Saunders, London, pp. 193–212.

Janota, I. and Smith, P. G. (1966), Adenomyoma in the pylorus. *Gut*, **7**, 194–199.

Järvinen, H., Nyberg, M. and Peltokallio, P. (1983), Upper gastrointestinal tract polyps in familial adenomatosis coli. *Gut*, **24**, 333–339.

Johansen, A. A. and Hart Hansen, O. (1973), Macroscopically demonstrable heterotopic gastric mucosa in the duodenum. *Scand. J. Gastroenterol.*, **8**, 59–63.

Kaneko, H., Yanaihara, N., Ito, S. *et al.* (1979), Somatostatinoma of the duodenum. *Cancer*, **44**, 2273–2279.

Kepes, J. J. and Zacharias, D. L. (1971), Gangliocytic paragangliomas of the duodenum. A report of two cases with light and electron microscopic examination. *Cancer*, **27**, 61–70.

Kreuning, J., Bosman, F. T., Kuiper, G. *et al.* (1978), Gastric and duodenal mucosa in 'healthy' individuals. An endoscopic and histopathological study of 50 volunteers. *J. Clin. Pathol.*, **31**, 69–77.

Lasser, A. and Koufman, W. B. (1977), Adenomyoma of the stomach. *Dig. Dis.*, **22**, 965–969.

Lessells, A. M. and Martin, D. F. (1982), Heterotopic gastric mucosa in the duodenum. *J. Clin. Pathol.*, **35**, 591–595.

Maratka, Z., Kocianova, J., Kudrmann, J. *et al.* (1979), Hyperplasia of Brunner's glands. Radiology, endoscopy and biopsy findings in 11 cases of diffuse, nodular and adenomatous form. *Acta Hepato-Gastroenterol.*, **26**, 64–69.

Martin, E. D. and Potet, F. (1974), Pathology of endocrine tumours of the GI tract. *Clin. Gastroenterol.*, **3**, 511–532.

Melmed, R. N. and Bouchier, I. A. D. (1972), Duodenal involvement in Gardner's syndrome. *Gut*, **13**, 524–527.

Mingazzini, P. L., Albedi, F. M. and Blandamura, V. (1982), Villous adenoma of the duodenum: cellular composition and histochemical findings. *Histopathology*, **6**, 235–244.

Miyawaki, E. H. and Straehley, C. J. (1973), Mucoceles of Brunner's glands. *Am. J. Surg.*, **126**, 688–690.

Nickels, J. and Laasonen, E. M. (1970), Pancreatic heterotopia. *Scand. J. Gastroenterol.*, **5**, 639–640.

O'Driscoll, B. R. C., Stevens, F. M., O'Gorman, T. A. *et al.* (1982), HLA type of patients with coeliac disease and malignancy in the west of Ireland. *Gut*, **23**, 662–665.

Ochsner, A. and Kleckner, M. S. Jr (1957), Primary malignant neoplasms of the duodenum. *J. Am. Med. Assoc.*, **163**, 413–417.

Olurin, E. O. and Solanke, T. F. (1968), Case of leiomyosarcoma of the duodenum and a review of the literature. *Gut*, **9**, 672–677.

Osborne, R., Toffler, R. and Lowman, R. M. (1973), Brunner's gland adenoma of the duodenum. *Dig. Dis.*, **18**, 689–694.

Ott, D. J., Wu, W. C., Shiflett, D. W. and Pennell, T. C. (1980), Inflammatory fibroid polyp of the duodenum. *Am. J. Gastroenterol.*, **73**, 62–64.

Paimela, H., Tallgren, L. G., Stenman, S. *et al.* (1984), Multiple duodenal polyps in uraemia: a little known clinical entity. *Gut*, **25**, 259–263.

Perzin, K. H. and Bridge, M. F. (1981), Adenomas of the small intestine: a clinicopathologic review of 51 cases and a study of their relationship to carcinoma. *Cancer*, **48**, 799–819.

Pomerantz, M. and Waldmann, T. A. (1963), Systemic lymphatic abnormalities associated with gastrointestinal protein loss secondary to intestinal lymphangiectasia. *Gastroenterology*, **45**, 703–711.

Rambaud, J-C. (1983), Small intestinal lymphomas and alpha-chain disease. *Clin. Gastroenterol.*, **12**, 743–766.

Rambaud, J-C. and Seligmann, M. (1976), Alpha-chain disease. *Clin. Gastroenterol.*, **5**, 341–358.

Ranzi, T., Castagnone, D., Velio, P. *et al.* (1981), Gastric and duodenal polyps in familial polyposis coli. *Gut*, **22**, 363–367.

Robertson, D. A. F., Dixon, M. F., Scott, B. B. *et al.* (1983), Small intestinal ulceration: diagnostic difficulties in relation to coeliac disease. *Gut*, **24**, 565–574.

Roggli, V. L., Judge, D. M. and McGavran, M. H. (1979), Duodenal glucagonoma: a case report. *Hum. Pathol.*, **10**, 350–353.

Schulten, M. F. Jr., Oyasu, R. and Beal, J. M. (1976), Villous adenoma of the duodenum. A case report and review of the literature. *Am. J. Surg.*, **132**, 90–96.

Shilkin, K. B., Zerman, B. J. and Blackwell, J. B. (1968), Lymphangiectatic cysts of the small bowel. *J. Pathol. Bacteriol.*, **96**, 353–358.

Spiller, R. C., Shousha, S. and Barrison, I. G. (1982), Heterotopic gastric tissue in the duodenum. A report of eight cases. *Dig. Dis. Sci*, **27**, 880–883.

Stokes, J. F., Turnberg, L. A. and Hawksley, J. C. (1964), Hyperplasia of Brunner's glands. *Gut*, **5**, 459–462.

Swinson, C. M., Hall, P. J., Bedford, P. A. and Booth, C. C. (1983), HLA antigens in coeliac disease associated with malignancy. *Gut*, **24**, 925–928.

Taylor, H. B. and Helwig, E. B. (1962), Benign nonchromaffin paragangliomas of the duodenum. *Virchows Arch. Pathol. Anat.*, **335**, 356–366.

Taylor, T. V. and Torrance, H. B. (1974), Haemangiomas of the gastrointestinal tract. *Br. J. Surg.*, **61**, 236–238.

Wald, A. and Milligan, F. D. (1975), The role of fiberoptic endoscopy in the diagnosis and management of duodenal neoplasms. *Dig. Dis.*, **20**, 499–505.

Whitehead, R. (1968), Primary lymphadenopathy complicating idiopathic steatorrhoea. *Gut*, **9**, 569–575.

Wilander, E., Grimelius, L., Lundqvist, G. and Skoog, V. (1979), Polypeptide hormones in argentaffin and argyrophil gastroduodenal endocrine tumors. *Am. J. Pathol.*, **96**, 519–530.

Williams, C. B., Goldblatt, M. and Delaney, P. V. (1982), 'Top and tail endoscopy' and follow-up in Peutz-Jeghers syndrome. *Endoscopy*, **14**, 82–84.

Wolk, D. P., Knapper, W. H. and Farr, G. H. (1973), Brunner's gland cystadenoma of the duodenum. *Am. J. Surg.*, **126**, 439–440.

Yao, T., Iida, M., Ohsato, K. *et al.* (1977), Duodenal lesions in familial polyposis of the colon. *Gastroenterology*, **73**, 1086–1092.

Yassinger, S., Imperato, T. J., Midgley, R. Jr. *et al.* (1977), Leiomyosarcoma of the duodenum. *Gastrointest. Endosc.*, **24**, 38–40.

Zarling, E. J. (1981), Gastric adenomyoma with coincidental pancreatic rest: a case report. *Gastrointest. Endosc.*, **27**, 175–177.

13 Miscellaneous conditions of the upper gastrointestinal tract

13.1 Oesophageal webs and rings

Oesophageal webs consist of single, or less commonly multiple, thin mucosal membranes which project into the oesophageal lumen. They can occur at all levels but are most common in the postcricoid region where they are usually attached anteriorly and laterally and have an eccentric lumen posteriorly. A significant proportion of upper oesophageal webs have been in women with glossitis and iron deficiency anaemia, the Plummer-Vinson syndrome (Shamma'a and Benedict, 1958). Webs may also occur in association with skin disorders such as benign mucous membrane pemphigus and epidermolysis bullosa. Others have followed ingestion of irritants or occurred in reflux oesophagitis and some are probably congenital.

Histological appearances show normal squamous epithelium or there may be acanthosis and para-or hyperkeratosis. Marked basal cell hyperplasia and elongation of submucosal papillae in biopsies from all levels of the oesophagus have been described in two patients with multiple oesophageal webs (Janisch and Eckardt, 1982). There is a significant association between the presence of oesophageal webs and the development of carcinoma of the buccal mucosa or oesophagus and in the series reported by Shamma'a and Benedict (1958) this occurred in 9 of 58 patients.

Mucosal rings at the lower end of the oesophagus, consisting of a symmetrical concentric transverse fold of mucosa projecting into the lumen, are not uncommon at autopsy (Goyal et al., 1971) or endoscopy (Arvanitakis, 1977). A sliding hiatus hernia is often present as well. The majority of patients are asymptomatic but dysphagia may develop with decreasing diameter of the lumen. Histological studies have in general shown that the upper surface of the ring consists of normal squamous epithelium and the lower surface of junctional epithelium (Section 2.2.2).

13.2   Amyloidosis

The gastrointestinal tract is a common and early site of involvement in both primary and secondary generalized amyloidosis (Gilat *et al.*, 1969), and if suspected the rectum is the preferred biopsy site. In the occasional case where the rectal biopsy is negative yet there is a strong clinical suspicion of amyloid, gastric or small intestinal biopsies should be taken. Even though commonly affected definite clinical signs and symptoms referable to this site are unusual. When they are present endoscopy can show thickening of the gastric folds with discrete areas of haemorrhage (Coughlin *et al.*, 1980). Massive infiltration may give an appearance resembling a diffusely spreading carcinoma (Shnider and Burka, 1955). In such cases the presence of amyloid may be obvious in the lamina propria of the mucosa (Fig. 13.1) associated with capillaries, and in submucosal blood vessels. In other situations it is only apparent after the use of confirmatory special stains, and for routine use on formalin-fixed material

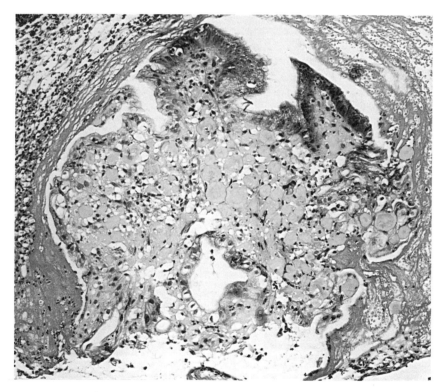

Fig. 13.1   Amyloid. Circumscribed nodules fill the lamina propria of this gastric biopsy. HE × 150.

a metachromatic stain such as crystal violet and the Sirius Red method with polarized light are recommended (Tribe and Perry, 1979).

13.3   Cytomegalovirus infection

As well as affecting the newborn, cytomegalovirus (CMV) infection may also occur in adults most of whom are immunologically deficient as a result of diseases such as leukaemia or lymphoma or following the use of immunosuppressive drugs. Some cases have occurred after blood trans-fusion and a few have been in apparently healthy individuals. Gastro-intestinal involvement has mostly been documented in surgical or autopsy material (Henson, 1972). In a recent biopsy study of patients undergoing renal transplantation (Franzin et al., 1981) CMV inclusions were identified post-operatively in approximately half, occurring particu-larly in the Brunner's glands of the duodenal bulb but also in the glands and lamina propria of the gastric mucosa. An accompanying rise in antibody titre to CMV was present in this group and the use of azathio-prine was considered to be a major factor in the development of infection.

The typical inclusions which occur in greatly enlarged cells are intranuclear and separated from the nuclear membrane by a wide halo. Less commonly basophilic, PAS positive, cytoplasmic inclusions are present (Figs 13.2 and 13.3). The cytoplasmic membrane of infected cells is accentuated. Inclusions associated with gastric ulcers have occurred in fibroblasts within granulation tissue and in endothelial cells of small blood vessels as well as in glandular mucosal cells at the ulcer margins (Henson, 1972; Campbell et al., 1977).

13.4   Gastric xanthelasma

These lesions, also known as lipid islands, have been noted at endoscopy in 0.4 to 6.3% of non-operated patients (Domellöf et al., 1977; Terruzzi et al., 1980), but their prevalence is higher in patients with a gastric stump, increasing with length of follow-up. Thus in one series 60% of patients had lesions 23 years after a Billroth II resection (Domellöf et al., 1977).

Macroscopically they appear as yellow or orange, clearly demarcated macules with a somewhat irregular outline, mostly 1–2 mm in diameter and rarely exceeding 5 mm, which occur preferentially in the antrum and related to the lesser curve in non-operated subjects, and close to the stoma, on the posterior wall, or along the greater curvature in operated patients. Larger lesions may be nodular and protrude above the surface (McCaffery, 1975). Xanthelasma may be single or multiple but rarely exceed ten in number.

Histologically, a focal group of foam cells is present in the lamina

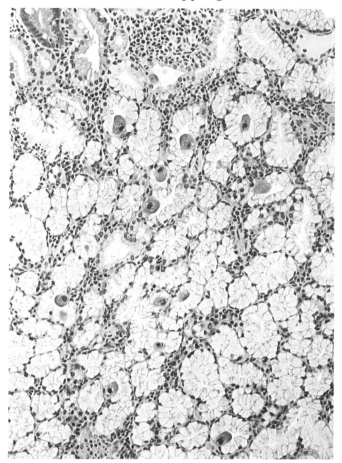

Fig. 13.2 Numerous epithelial cells of Brunner's glands show evidence of cytomegalovirus infection in this duodenal biopsy from a renal transplant recipient. HE × 150.

propria, predominantly in the superficial parts of the mucosa (Fig. 13.4). Individual cells are polygonal or rounded with distinct cell outlines and from 10–30 μm in diameter. The cytoplasm has a distinctive fine mesh-like network with vacuoles from one to several microns in diameter, outlined by remnants of fine eosinophilic cytoplasm. The nucleus is small, round or oval and central, or slightly eccentric. No mitoses or atypia are present (Fig. 13.5). Inflammatory cells are scanty or absent although adjacent mucosa often shows gastritis, sometimes with atrophy and intestinal metaplasia.

The most important distinction in practice is from infiltrating carcinoma

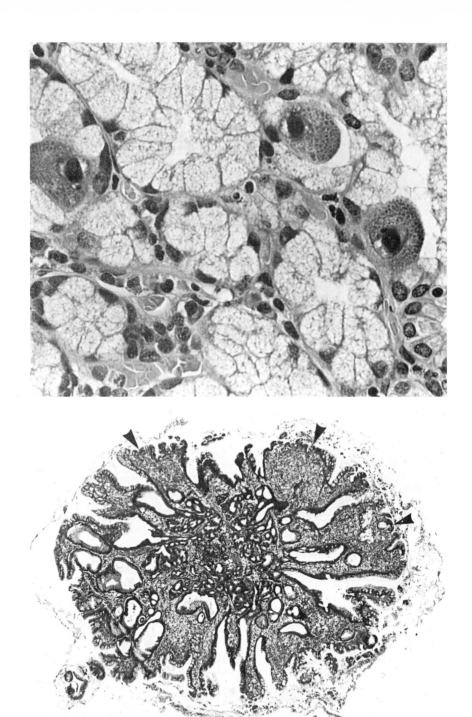

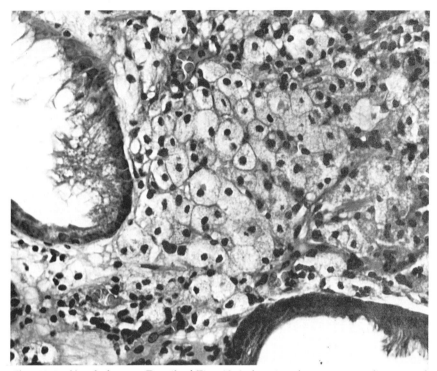

Fig. 13.5 Xanthelasma. Detail of Fig. 13.4 showing foamy macrophages with bland, centrally sited nuclei. HE × 375.

of signet-ring and other mucin-secreting varieties (Heilmann, 1973), particularly in the setting of the post-operative stomach where there is an increased risk of malignancy. I have seen examples where xanthelasma has been diagnosed as a mucocellular carcinoma, and the opposite situation when a small collection of carcinoma cells in a biopsy has been interpreted as a lipid island. Apart from the endoscopic appearances, when present, and the cytological features described above the use of a periodic acid Schiff/alcian blue (PAS/AB) stain is very helpful in differentiating the two, as carcinoma cells will stain strongly due to their content of either PAS or alcian blue positive mucin (not infrequently a mixture), whereas foam cells are unstained or only faintly PAS positive. Foam cells are also sudanophilic. In my experience focal collections of mucin-containing macrophages (muciphages) are extremely uncommon in

Fig. 13.3   Detail of Fig. 13.2 shows intranuclear inclusions with surrounding halo together with granular cytoplasmic inclusions in three infected cells. HE × 600.
Fig. 13.4   Xanthelasma. In this gastric biopsy groups of large round cells are filling and expanding the lamina propria (arrowed). HE × 38.

gastric biopsy material and are easily distinguished from carcinoma cells by their low nuclear/cytoplasmic ratio and the bland appearance of their centrally located and pyknotic-appearing nuclei (Fig. 8.18).

The pathogenesis of these lesions is unclear. Chemical analysis has shown the presence of cholesterol in all and of neutral fat in one third (Kimura et al., 1969). The association with chronic gastritis and intestinal metaplasia and their frequency in the operated stomach suggests that biliary reflux is an important aetiological factor. Ultrastructural studies have shown that the foam cells originate from two sources, histiocytes and smooth muscle cells (Böger and Hort, 1977).

References

Arvanitakis, C. (1977), Lower esophageal ring: endoscopic and therapeutic aspects. Gastrointest. Endosc., **24**, 17–18.

Böger, A. and Hort, W. (1977), The importance of smooth muscle cells in the development of foam cells in the gastric mucosa. An electron microscopic study. Virchows Arch. Path. Anat., **372**, 287–297.

Campbell, D. A., Piercey, J. R. A., Shnitka, T. K. et al. (1977), Cytomegalovirus-associated gastric ulcer. Gastroenterology, **72**, 533–535.

Coughlin, G. P., Reiner, R. G. and Grant, A. K. (1980), Endoscopic diagnosis of amyloidosis. Gastrointest. Endosc., **26**, 154–155.

Domellöf, L., Eriksson, S., Helander, H. F. and Janunger, K-G. (1977), Lipid islands in the gastric mucosa after resection for benign ulcer disease. Gastroenterology, **72**, 14–18.

Franzin, G., Muolo, A. and Griminelli, T. (1981), Cytomegalovirus inclusions in the gastroduodenal mucosa of patients after renal transplantation. Gut, **22**, 698–701.

Gilat, T., Revach, M. and Sohar, E. (1969), Deposition of amyloid in the gastrointestinal tract. Gut, **10**, 98–104.

Goyal, R. K., Bauer, J. L. and Spiro, H. M. (1971), The nature and location of lower esophageal ring. N. Engl. J. Med., **284**, 1175–1180.

Heilmann, K. (1973), Lipid islands in gastric mucosa. Beitr. Pathol., **149**, 411–419.

Henson, D. (1972), Cytomegalovirus inclusion bodies in the gastrointestinal tract. Arch. Pathol., **93**, 477–482.

Janisch, H. D. and Eckardt, V. F. (1982), Histological abnormalities in patients with multiple esophageal webs. Dig. Dis. Sci., **27**, 503–506.

Kimura, K., Hiramoto, T. and Buncher, C. R. (1969), Gastric xanthelasma. Arch. Pathol., **87**, 110–117.

McCaffery, T. D. Jr. (1975), Xanthomas of the stomach. Gastrointest. Endosc., **21**, 167–168.

Shnider, B. I. and Burka, P. (1955), Amyloid disease of the stomach simulating gastric carcinoma. Gastroenterology, **28**, 424–430.

Shamma'a, M. H. and Benedict, E. B. (1958), Esophageal webs. A report of 58 cases and an attempt at classification. N. Engl. J. Med., **259**, 378–384.

Terruzzi, V., Minoli, G., Butti, G. C. and Rossini, A. (1980), Gastric lipid islands in the gastric stump and in non-operated stomach. Endoscopy, **12**, 58–62.

Tribe, C. R. and Perry, V. A. (1979), Diagnosis of amyloidosis. A.C.P. Broadsheet **92**, 1–11.

14 Cytology of the oesophagus, stomach and duodenum

O. A. N. HUSAIN

14.1 The development of gastrointestinal cytology

The advent of fibrescopes of increasing versatility and reducing size has revolutionized cytological diagnosis of lesions of the upper gastro-intestinal tract.

Until the late 1940s gastro-oesophageal cytology was restricted to simple aspirates or wash techniques when instruments in the form of sponges (Zelltopfsonde), brushes and abrasive balloons had a short vogue and the three-channel irrigation Faucher tube and Woods gastro-scope were introduced. The use of cytology by these techniques was more for screening and detection than for diagnosis, and it was not until the development of the flexible fibrescope that more purposive brush, suc-tion and directional lavage samples were collected from hitherto inaccess-ible sites (Kasugai, 1976; Winawer et al., 1976). This resulted in a better preserved and presentable cell sample and improved diagnostic accuracy (Kameya et al., 1964; Kasugai, 1964; Kidokoro et al., 1966; Liavag et al., 1971; Kasugai and Kobayashi, 1974; Winawer et al., 1976; Shida, 1976; Witzel et al., 1976). The history of improvement is reflected more in techniques than in time as seen from the long list of authors depicted in Table 14.1.

There was a significant improvement in the detection rate in Japan during the ten years from 1956 as shown by the rise in the proportion of early surface cancers from 3.8% to 34.5% of all cancers found (Prolla et al., 1969) due mainly to a combination of biopsy and directional wash cytology. It was of interest to note that the highest levels of detection by cytology of gastric cancer, with a sensitivity approaching 97% (Kasugai, 1968), occurred using a directional jet wash technique, though Halter et al. (1977) were only able to achieve a 50% accuracy. In fact, the Japanese were more enthusiastic about directional wash than brush samples and it was in the West that the latter found more favour and success.

Table 14.1 The efficiency of various authors using different sampling techniques

Series	No. with cancer	Accuracy (%)	Method
Papanicolaou and Cooper (1947)	27	37	Fasting aspirate
Graham, Ulfelder and Green (1948)	24	62	Fasting aspirate
Traut et al. (1952)	42	71	Papain lavage
Crozier, Middleton and Ross (1956)	29	69	Lavage and brush abrasion
Seybolt and Papanicolaou (1957)	114	66	Abrasive balloon
Fakuda (quoted by Tazaki, 1959)	76	85	Modified balloon
Cabre-Fiol et al. (1959)	94	90	Mandril-sound
Raskin, Kirsner and Palmer (1959)	131	95	Gastric washings
Schade (1960)	258	97	Gastric washings
Witte (1959)	184	65	Zelltopfsonde
MacDonald et al. (1963)	89	93	Chymotrypsin wash
Taebel, Prolla and Kirsner (1965)	282	81	Gastric washings
Blendis et al. (1967)	100	81	Gastric washings
Kasugai (1968)	375	97	Fibregastroscopic lavage
Shida (1971)	60	90	Fibregastroscopic brush
Witzel et al. (1976)	73	84	Fibrescopic brush
Thompson et al. (1977)	59	90	Fibrescopic brush
Young and Hughes (1977)	61	92	Fibrescopic brush
MacKenzie et al. (1977)		94	Fibrescopic brush
Boddington (1978)	84	79	Fibrescopic brush
Husain et al. (1980)	61	83	Fibrescopic brush

The use of the imprint smear technique (Yoshii *et al.*, 1970) to achieve cytological sampling of a deeper tissue plane was considered superior to that of directional washes (Tamura *et al.*, 1977) but the manipulation of this minute biopsy fragment can interfere with histological interpretation and its use for cytology has lost favour with many authorities. A series of good, deep plunges of the gastric brush into the mucosa can often be as effective in sampling cells from a depth equivalent to, or beyond, that of the bite of the small biopsy forceps, though the imprint has the virtue of reflecting the structural arrangement of the cells.

As sampling and preparation techniques are the main factors contributing to the accuracy of diagnosis, and as they are in the joint province of both gastroenterologist and pathologist some detail must be recorded here. It is paramount that a specially trained technician or nurse be involved in the production of these specimens.

14.1.1   *Simple blind aspirates or wash specimens*

This approach is still used in those cases unwilling or unable to undergo gastroscopy due to stenosis of the pharynx or oesophagus or in the screening mode, as it is only about a half to a third as expensive as the fibrescopic brush sample (Husain, 1976). Moreover, it may become the simpler mode of sampling for those more refined immunological or cytochemical techniques where more specific identification or functional assessment of cell behaviour can be achieved.

The oesophagus lends itself well to simple 20–40 ml direct washings by buffered saline above any stricture, though almost as much information can be derived from the collection of stomach contents beyond any lesion or stricture.

For gastric washings the patient needs to fast overnight, although encouraged to drink liberal supplies of water as dehydration will seriously restrict cell exfoliation. A Levin tube, plastic or rubber (12–14 F.G. or 3 – 4 mm diameter), with a few more holes cut out near its end for a broader salvage, is passed through the mouth or, preferably, via the nose, to a mid-gastric position, and the whole of the resting juice is aspirated and kept. About 250–300 ml of buffered saline is then introduced down the tube, after which the abdomen is massaged and the patient made to flex and extend the body so as to induce exfoliation of the surface mucosal cells. This washing is then aspirated when the procedure may be repeated. If much tenacious mucus is present it may be necessary to repeat the test by giving the patient 7 mg of alphachymotrypsin in a glass of water half-an-hour before the gastric wash, which is then performed using a further 7 mg of alphachymotrypsin in a sodium acetate buffer, pH 5.6. At this pH the enzyme digests the mucus but not the mucosal cells.

The resting juice and each gastric wash are immediately neutralized by N/10 sodium hydroxide, if necessary to pH 6, but not beyond, as alkali destroys cells quicker than acid, and the samples centrifuged rapidly, preferably in ice cold siliconized tubes. The deposit is smeared on to about six clean slides some of which are wet-fixed for Papanicolaou staining, and a few thinner smears rapidly air dried for staining by a Romanowsky technique (e.g. May-Gruenwald-Giemsa schedule). The screening and checking of such smears calls for much skill and patience in the interpretation of cell changes, which are by no means as clear-cut or as florid as brush samples.

14.1.2   Fibrescopic brush and directional wash samples

There are only a few major manufacturers of fibrescopes but we have used the Olympus instruments, either the GFD end-viewing one for the oesophagus, or side-viewing one for the stomach. The more versatile, oblique viewing instrument with its ability to move through 180° has, however become the model of choice as it can be used for both stomach and oesophagus, while the smaller paediatric version is welcomed by adults as more acceptable and still provides an effective instrument, albeit with smaller biopsy samples. The schedule is common to that used to collect a tissue biopsy for histology, in fact it is becoming the custom to collect both samples in most instances.

After fasting overnight the patient is sedated with diazepam intravenously and the larynx anaesthetized with 1% lignocaine. The saline or glycerol-lubricated fibrescope (oily lubricants may obscure cellular detail) is passed with the patient lying in the supine or left-lateral position, with or without an airway. After inspection of the stomach any lesion is photographed and both brush and biopsy samples are taken. It is preferable to obtain the brush sample before the biopsy as the latter results in bleeding which both obscures the lesion and detracts from the quality of the cytological sample, whereas interpretation of the biopsy is not affected by this order of collection (Thompson *et al.*, 1977).

(a) *Collection of brush and wash specimens.* The collection of a good brush sample usually requires an experienced assistant as the gastroscopist may well be engaged in manoeuvring the end of the scope and holding the lesion in focus while the assistant can be free to manipulate the brush. The need then is to plunge the brush firmly and briskly into the mucosa five to ten times so that the lamina propria is penetrated. Anything less than this fails to obtain a reliable sample and may lead to a false negative result. The site and mode of sampling is important as will be seen from Fig. 14.1. Here the need to sample from the growing outer edge of a cavitating ulcer is logical, but the areas to sample in the various forms of surface cancer are just as important, as is the need to sample straight down into the centre of a possibly tumorous shallow ulcer when there is a suspicion of a mesodermal tumour. The commonest of these are leiomyosarcoma or lymphoma. Penetration to a depth sufficient to retrieve deeper cell tissue is then paramount.

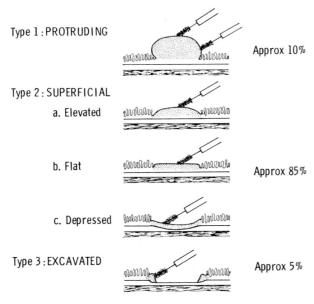

Type 1 : PROTRUDING

Approx 10%

Type 2 : SUPERFICIAL

a. Elevated

b. Flat

Approx 85%

c. Depressed

Type 3 : EXCAVATED

Approx 5%

Fig. 14.1 Mode of sampling by gastric brush from early and surface cancers of the stomach and their approximate incidence in Japan.

Originally, the large and robust brush issued by the makers for cleansing the endoscope was used, but this resulted in the restricted practice of using the brush as the last act of a gastroscopy and withdrawing it within the instrument before removing the latter from the patient. Pulling the brush right through the fibrescope channel left most of the material inside the endoscope. Such a brush is still worthwhile when used to sample the more stenotic oesophageal lesions, but nowadays there are ranges of smaller brushes enclosed inside transparent Teflon sheaths which permit multiple samples to be collected. The brush sample, when obtained, is pulled back just within the Teflon sheath and the whole sheath is withdrawn. In Japan and in many centres in the United States and Europe up to ten specimens of both biopsy and brush samples are collected, but in the United Kingdom such practices are not followed. Here one, perhaps two, cytology samples are collected for examination.

Directional wash samples are not often collected outside Japan but the technique is simple. The opening of a Teflon tube is directed at a particular lesion at close quarters and forceful injection of buffered saline is aimed at the site. Immediate suction by the syringe injecting the fluid results in salvage of cells from that area.

(b) *Preparation of brush and wash samples.* Ideally, brush smears should be made immediately but the brush head, if withdrawn just within the Teflon tube, will maintain reasonable cell morphology for 15–30 min so that the specimen can be rapidly transported to the laboratory where more ideal conditions for processing exist with minimal loss of technician time. The brush is first protruded from the Teflon tube over a small one ounce bottle ('universal container') containing about 10 ml of buffered saline. Any drop of fluid containing cells is thus not lost. The brush is then rolled rather than rubbed on to a clean glass slide. About four to six, or even more, smears can be made from each brush sample, most of which are rapidly wet-fixed in alcohol for Papanicolaou staining whilst one or two of the thinner and later-made smears are rapidly air dried for staining by a Romanowsky stain (May-Gruenwald-Giemsa in our laboratories).

Even after making this number of direct smears the brush retains a considerable amount of cells and these can be agitated off by a simple vortexer with the brush head immersed in the vial containing buffered saline. Care should be taken during vortexing to avoid any droplet spray being transmitted to the atmosphere by the simple procedure of inserting a cotton wool plug into the mouth of the vial. In fact, full protective procedures with mask, gown and gloves should be mandatory for staff preparing such specimens, as even rolling a brush on a slide creates small droplet particles in the surrounding air. This sample is then aspirated on to a Millipore filter, fixed in alcohol and stained by the Papanicolaou technique. This often displays a remarkable amount of cells and occasionally may be the best if not the only evidence of neoplasia.

The brushes are sold as disposable but can, with care after total immersion in 2% gluteraldehyde overnight, be thoroughly and safely cleansed with the tip of a needle or another firm nylon brush, sweeping towards the tip of the wire under running water, then sterilized by formalin steam at 70–80°C for 4–6 hours. In this way, and with microscopic inspection of the bristle ends, these tiny fragile brushes can be re-used up to ten or more times. As labour costs go up, if the price of the mass produced brush comes down, this exercise may well cease to be cost-effective, but it is a regular part of the cytology department's responsibilities to ensure removal of any residual material and to preserve the tiny brush heads as long as possible.

Directional wash samples can either be concentrated in a similar fashion to the blind tube wash specimen by centrifuging in ice-cold siliconized tubes or aspirated onto a Millipore membrane, or both techniques can be employed. For smaller fluid samples cyto-centrifuge specimens can be made.

14.2   The cytology of oesophageal, gastric and duodenal specimens

As each of these sites produces distinctive cell patterns and problems in diagnosis they will be dealt with separately.

It can be said by way of introduction that not all that is seen in the smears necessarily originates from the organ in question, as both the upper and lower respiratory tract and the bucco-pharyngeal regions give rise to much swallowed material that will appear in oesophageal or gastric samples, and this must always be remembered when interpreting such smears. Perhaps the most common 'foreign' cell is the buccal squame which is usually of a fairly mature intermediate type, though both parabasal and superficial cells occur. The other common and distinctive cell is the pulmonary macrophage which, with its ingested black carbon or brown blood pigment, should present no difficulty in interpretation. With the wash samples, other contaminants, such as food particles (mostly vegetable and sometimes meat fibre), dental powder and other ingested material serve to obscure the cytological picture, as do the columnar cells, mucus and polymorphs that may well derive from the respiratory tract. On the whole, the brush samples do not suffer from these contaminants so much, and preservation of the cells is much better than in wash specimens. In fact, it is important to know which type of preparation one is examining in both pulmonary and gastrointestinal tract samples as the appearances differ considerably. The washed-off sheets of gastric cells, having been in contact with saline during the process time, lose quite a lot of cellular detail compared with the fresher cells brushed from the intact mucosa. Here, the chromatin looks more active and the nucleoli more distinct and there is a greater temptation to overcall a lesion as neoplastic.

14.2.1   Oesophageal cell samples

(a) *Benign lesions of the oesophagus.* These consist mainly of those from a reflux oesophagitis where squames, mostly of the mature variety, show inflammatory changes of varying degree. There is increased nuclear size and density with a relatively uniform chromatin pattern and disturbed granular (sometimes vacuolated) cytoplasm, staining polychromatically with the Papanicolaou stain and sometimes containing engulfed polymorphs. In fact, such intra-cytoplasmic polymorphs and cell debris appear to be more common in benign than in malignant lesions of the oesophagus.

What causes difficulties is the presence of the deep or parabasal squames, originally described by Gephart and Graham (1959), but these usually show good cellular adhesion in contrast to the malignant variety, though even here syncytia occur. Another, but rare, condition is herpetic oesophagitis with large, immature-looking cells showing multinucleation and intranuclear inclusions which can cause some concern when seen in benign lesions (Lasser, 1977). This condition may be associated with neoplasia (Berg, 1955).

(b) *Malignant lesions of the oesophagus.* These are predominantly squamous cell carcinomas and are easily recognized by the bizarre, brightly-staining red or orange keratinized squamous cells in association with less well differentiated but obvious cancer cells with their large, irregular hyperchromatic nuclei. It is only when poorly differentiated malignant cells are present that the distinction between squamous and glandular cancer becomes difficult (Figs 14.2 and 14.3). At times this makes interpretation almost impossible as syncytial forms of squamous cancer can confuse the

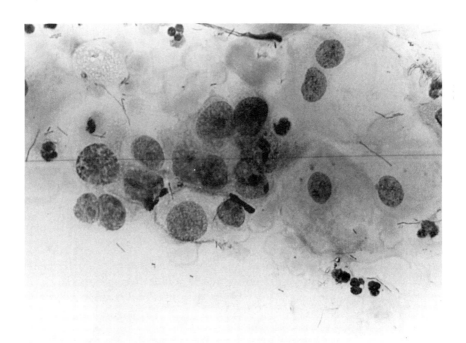

Fig. 14.2   A well-differentiated squamous cancer of oesophagus. PAP × 160.

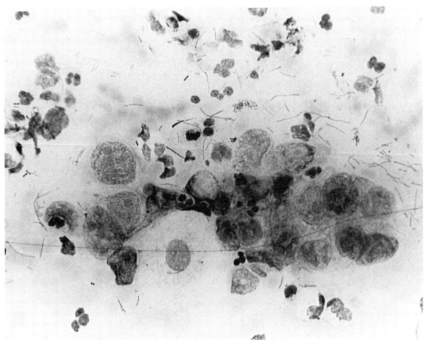

Fig. 14.3   A poorly differentiated squamous cancer of oesophagus. PAP × 160.

picture. In such cases the multiple and more angular nucleoli and the tendency to form concentric rings in the perinuclear cytoplasm point more to squamous neoplasia compared with the usually solitary, large central nucleoli in the eccentrically positioned nuclei and the more frothy cytoplasm characteristically seen in glandular tumour cells.

14.2.2   Gastric cell samples

(a) *Benign conditions of the stomach.* These consist of regenerative gastric polyps, chronic atrophic gastritis with intestinal metaplasia and benign peptic ulcers (Figs 14.4 and 14.5).

It is difficult to make a diagnosis of a gastric polyp on cytological grounds although in some cases polypoid fragments of mucosa occur in smears. The identification of atrophic gastritis, however, is relatively easy and important as it is in such cases that 70 to 80% of gastric carcinomas arise. It is fortunate here that the destructive mineral acid is absent and only the organic acids from cell and bacterial metabolism exist at pH 5 to 6 with much increase in mucus which tends to preserve cellular detail. Essentially, the mucosa is chronically inflamed with a resultant excessive

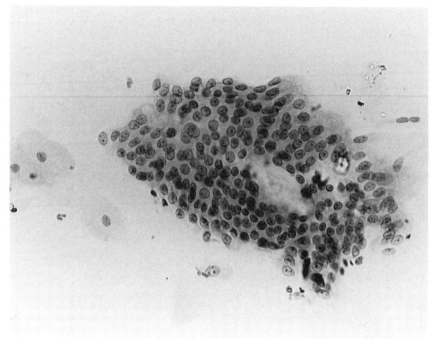

Fig. 14.4   A sheet of benign gastric mucosal cells. PAP × 40.

spontaneous exfoliation of single cells and large and small sheets. The cells reflect an atrophy, intestinal metaplasia and increased mucus secretion. There is a general rounding up of the columnar cells, some nuclear crowding and an increase in nuclear chromatin, though this is relatively uniform, albeit sometimes with nucleoli (Fig. 14.5). These, though sometimes prominent, are not large in size and the general cohesion of the sheet of cells indicates the benign nature of the condition. The concomitant increase in mucin-secreting cells (goblet cells) produces a more rounded cell with the nucleus being displaced to the side of the cell by the mucous globule. This gives rise to the so-called signet ring in its extreme form. Intestinalization of the mucosa – mainly in the pyloric antrum – gives rise to a larger, darker columnar cell with a more central, enlarged and hyperchromatic nucleus, be the cell still columnar, flattened or globular. All this presents a characteristic picture associated with a chronic inflammatory exudate of polymorphs, lymphocytes and plasma cells. The extreme reactivity seen at times in atrophic gastritis (as also with repairing or regenerating epithelium from a healing ulcer) often presents considerable difficulty in deciding between reactivity and neoplasia (Fig. 14.6). Here the nucleolar size is small and the nuclear–nucleolar ratio

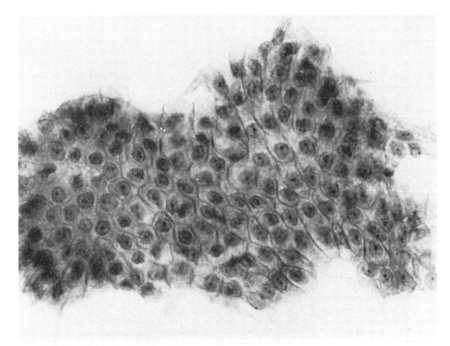

Fig. 14.5 Active gastric mucosal cells. Note prominent nucleoli but uniformity of nuclei. PAP × 100.

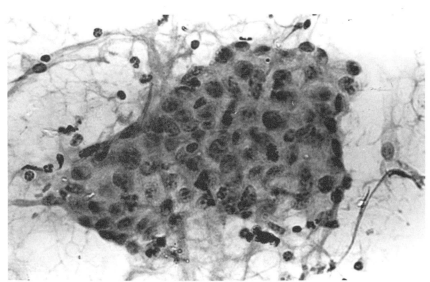

Fig. 14.6 Markedly reactive sheet of gastric mucosal cells. Note mitoses. PAP × 100.

remains usually between 15 : 1 and 20 : 1, while malignant cells usually display a ratio around 10 : 1. Danno (1976) has quantified this finding and with a formula has presented good evidence of the value of this feature. The cells still appear to retain their cytoplasmic edges and though the cell pattern is disturbed there is still a degree of uniformity and cell cohesion.

The presence of inflammatory cells which are mostly polymorphs with some histiocytes and (if the lymphoid follicles are enlarged) an increase of active lymphocytes, both mature and transformed and sometimes cleaved with some mitoses, together with some larger histiocytes containing ingested, hyperchromatic pink and purplish particles (tingible bodies) serves to make the diagnosis difficult for the inexperienced (Hughes *et al.*, 1978).

(b) *Malignant lesions of the stomach.* These consist predominantly of adenocarcinomas of varying degrees of differentiation (Figs 14.7, 14.8 and 14.9), though sarcomas (Cabre-Fiol *et al.*, 1975) and malignant lymphomas

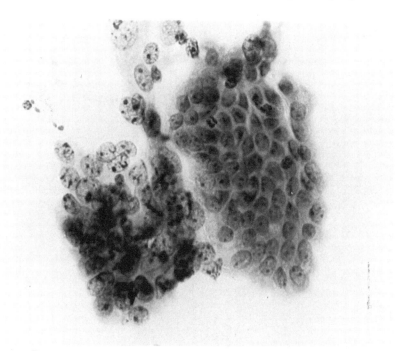

Fig. 14.7 Benign gastric mucosa and early well-differentiated surface cancer (in same smear). PAP × 100.

Fig. 14.8 Well-differentiated polypoid adenocarcinoma of stomach. PAP × 160.
Fig. 14.9 Poorly differentiated adenocarcinoma of the stomach. PAP × 160.

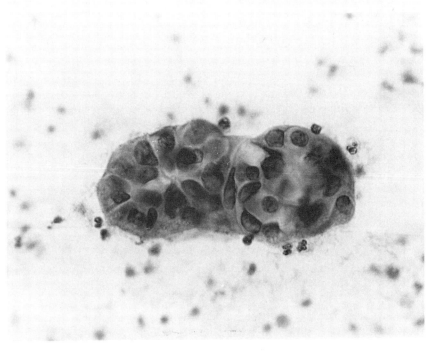

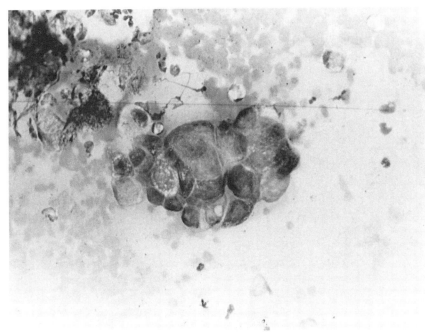

(Kline and Goldstein, 1974; Prolla *et al.*, 1977) are being diagnosed with increasing accuracy. As with glandular cancer elsewhere the pattern varies both with type and differentiation. Most well-differentiated tumours will demonstrate significant alteration from the columnar pattern with anisonucleosis and varying degrees of chromasia, many cancer cells being quite pale with fine granular chromatin pattern and occasionally almost bland, right up to the hyperchromatic nucleus with marked dyskaryosis, that is, with irregular chromatin condensation occurring characteristically beneath the nuclear membrane and around the prominent nucleoli as well as within the nucleoplasm. It is the nuclear–nucleolar ratio of around 10 or less that provides the most valuable characteristic of neoplasia (Danno, 1976).

Other features such as an increased nuclear–cytoplasmic ratio may not be evident in the more differentiated tumours, and the loss of cytoplasmic margins is so commonly seen in benign gastric lesions that it gives little support to the diagnosis of malignancy. The cells form irregular clusters and morulae with nuclei that marginate around the cell edge, and a bluish brown mucoid secretion may exist in the cytoplasm. A variant of less well-differentiated tumour occurs as palely staining sheets with bluish floccular or granular cytoplasm and fairly monomorphic, rounded nuclei with prominent nucleoli. As the tumour appears less differentiated the cells become more bizarre, the pattern pleomorphic and disaggregated with an increasing nuclear–cytoplasmic ratio, a more dyskaryotic nucleoplasm and with more prominent nucleoli. Mitoses are frequent and there is more degenerative change and necrosis present. It is the lack of cell cohesion that is the most marked characteristic of the grade of tumour (Young and Hughes, 1977).

Occasionally the tumour shows little in the way of nucleoli, a more bland nucleoplasm, perhaps multiple small and irregular chromocentres and produces palely staining spheres or morulae of tumour cells with nuclei in flat appliqué formation with the edge of the cytoplasmic mass similar to that seen in some metastases from breast carcinoma in serous fluids.

Cytologically there is little to distinguish a surface cancer from a more advanced one other than perhaps a greater degree of inflammatory and degenerative change in the latter variety (Fig. 14.10). In the need to find such lesions, widespread and multiple brush samples should be collected or a wash technique used to obtain a wider salvage of cells. Examining the excised stomach for surface cancers may create a problem if neoplasia has been diagnosed by brush or wash cytology. It is believed by some that up to 10% of benign ulcers may have surface cancer somewhere in the adjacent mucosa and looking for this either by the elaborate and cumbersome giant Swiss roll technique of sectioning strips of stomach wall

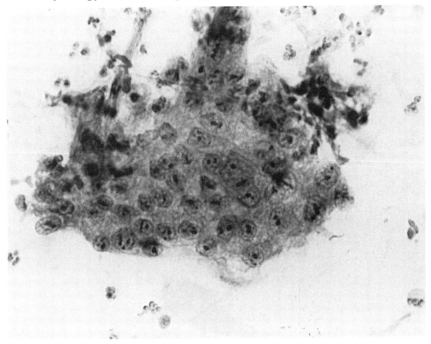

Fig. 14.10   A brush smear from a surface cancer of the stomach. PAP × 100.

(Mason, 1965) or by examination of multiple sections or of imprint or scrape smears from geographic sites on the mucosa may occasionally be necessary.

The uncommon carcinoma simplex or leather bottle stomach presents greater cytological problems if the brush is not made to penetrate the surface mucosa. A similar problem exists in diagnosing sarcomas and lymphoreticular tumours. It is essential that wherever such tumours as leiomyosarcomas and the lymphomas are suspected the brush should be vigorously plunged into the centre of a sessile or even slightly domed centre of an ulcer so as to penetrate to an underlying mesodermal tumour. Here the use of the Romanowsky-stained preparation is invaluable in classifying the tumour and it is here also that such stains used on imprints of the micro-biopsies would appear justified so as to provide evidence of a micro-anatomical structure.

14.2.3   Duodenal lesions

As carcinoma is extremely rare in the duodenal mucosa, cytology is used largely to diagnose duodenitis and to recognize any specific causes, such as *Giardia lamblia*, where the characteristic parasites are easily identified. (Wright *et al.*, 1977).

There are, however, tumours from two other sites that are diagnosable by cytology, those from the pancreas and the biliary tract. It is possible to collect secretions from both organs by duodenal intubation following injections of secretin and then pancreozymin so as to stimulate secretions from the pancreas and biliary tract respectively, or to intubate and aspirate from the pancreatic duct, or insert a fine brush and so collect a cellular sample (Henning and Witte, 1970; Hatfield *et al.*, 1974). When this is accompanied by endoscopic retrograde cholangiopancreatography (ERCP) the overall diagnostic accuracy can be well into the upper 80% (Hatfield *et al.*, 1975).

Again, with malignant lymphoma when deep duodenal brushing or biopsy imprint smears are performed, accuracies from 70 to 80% can be achieved (Kline and Goldstein, 1974; Nelson and Lanza, 1974; Posner *et al.*, 1975).

14.2.4   *Reporting on smears*

Reporting of gastric and oesophageal cytology is both easy and difficult. The negative cases are often the more arduous to screen as a thorough search must be made for any atypical feature. On the other hand, a frankly malignant case shows up clearly and quickly and it does not take long to establish a fairly definitive diagnosis. Here the answer can often be obtained within an hour or two of collecting the specimen.

It is the marginal changes that create the problems and require an exhaustive study before a report can be made. This usually means a report delayed to the next day. A rapid reporting system is, however, appreciated as the gastroenterologist or surgeon can anticipate and arrange for the next move at a much earlier stage and the patient is kept in suspense for a much shorter time.

It is inevitable that categorization of case reports occurs in order to provide a communicative shorthand between pathologist and clinician and here we rely on a sort of Papanicolaou grading system for our own and our clinical colleague's usage, which has proved effective and meaningful.

Grade I. This denotes an adequate specimen showing no sign of malignancy.

Grade II. Here it is also benign, but is accompanied by substantial inflammatory changes in the epithelial cells, mainly reflected in the nuclei.

Grade IIR. We have devised this grade in order to heighten the suspicion of an inflammatory or reactive-like smear pattern where the changes are bordering on the neoplastic – a so-called borderline lesion. It refers to a markedly atypical picture, requiring a repeat (R) or at least a close follow-up by either brush or biopsy, or both.

Grade III. Here there are atypical and often dyskaryotic cells which are suspicious of a pre-neoplastic lesion, or even one of invasion, but there is insufficient evidence to provide a confident report.

Grade IV. Here malignancy is obvious and diagnostic and as it is impossible to distinguish a surface from an invasive cancer it refers to both grades of lesion.

Grade O. This denotes an inadequate or unsatisfactory sample which may exist on its own – a totally unsatisfactory and unreadable sample graded as 'O' – or as O(I), or O(II), or even as O(III) where the specimen, though inadequate and unreliable, is also rated as possessing abnormal cells amounting to the grade number in parenthesis. (It leaves open the possibility of a more severe lesion detectable from a more reliable sample.)

The written report should be presented in three parts. Our practice has been to present firstly a descriptive cytological report which is comprehensive, but admittedly not always understood by the non-cytologist; secondly, the intelligence from, or interpretation of, the findings given in histological terms; and thirdly to give a recommendation for further investigational procedure, should the diagnosis not be explicit, or the lesion be so suspect as to warrant follow-up. In other words, we do not restrict ourselves to a simple malignant or benign option, as the reactive and hyperplastic changes encountered, especially in the glandular lesions, may be so borderline that it would be as much a folly to ignore such changes as to overcall them. We therefore utilize the category IIR (mentioned above) with due circumspection but with a simple explanation of concern.

Table 14.2 shows that the cases from a four-year survey in Charing Cross and St Stephen's Hospitals have produced a scatter of grades, while Table 14.3 expresses the accuracies of both cytological and histological biopsies in a few published series. It will be evident that the cytological samples appear to be marginally more accurate and probably reflect the larger cellular samples more fully presented on slides from the brush, compared with the small histological biopsy sometimes with compression-distortion and not always sufficiently sectioned to express the full cellular content of the excised fragment.

It is the final column of Table 14.3 summating the accuracies of both samples that provides the more significant message and indicates the value of both techniques being used.

Table 14.2 Gastric and oesophageal brush cytology: Charing Cross and St Stephen's Hospital 1976–79. Incidence of lesions and accuracy of histological and cytological reports

Normal	Inflammatory	Atypical (to follow)	Susp. malig.	Malignant	Total
160(17)	285(14)	17(2)	19(2)	75	556

Unsatisfactory samples in parenthesis

Total cases	Pos. cytol. Pos. hist.	Pos. cytol. Neg. hist.	Neg. cytol. Pos. hist.	Pos. cytol. unsatisfac. biopsy	Pos. hist. unsatisfac. cytol.	False neg. both	False pos. both
110	70	11	9	11	7	1	1

Cytology sensitivity (overall)   92/110 = 83.6%
Cytology sensitivity (minus unsatis.)   92/103 = 89.3%
Histology sensitivity (overall)   86/110 = 78.1%
Histology sensitivity (minus unsatis.)   86/99 = 85.1%
Combined histology and cytology sensitivity   108/110 = 98.1%

Table 14.3 Percentage accuracy of endoscopic cytology and biopsy in the diagnosis of gastric tumours.

Author	Date	Total sample	Correct cytol.	Correct histol.	Correct combined
Kobayashi et al.	1970	26	97.0	66.7	100.0
Serck-Hanssen et al.	1973	68	94.1	52.9	94.1
Bemventui et al.	1975	58	77.8	82.2	?
Smithies et al.	1975	34	82.4	61.8	97.1
Witzel et al.	1976	73	83.6	79.5	95.9
Young and Hughes	1977	61	91.8	68.9	91.8
Boddington (incl. 1969/73 series)	1978	84	78.5	72.6	92.8
St Stephen's/Charing Cross series	1981	110	83.6	78.1	98.1

It can be seen that there has not been a false positive report in this particular series though we do have the IIR category that permits us an identity of an atypical borderline picture. This apparent underreporting, we feel, errs on the right side and seven of these cases turned out to be malignant by subsequent cytology or histology. Of course, we will not know fully what false negative results we have in either histology or cytology until cases have been followed for some years.

A review of the smears in the cytologically negative/histologically positive cases has not disclosed any atypical or malignant cells and one can only presume that sampling was at fault. Here, multiple biopsies and brushes would help to reduce such an error.

False positives have been reported by most authorities (Richards and Spriggs, 1961; Prolla *et al.*, 1977) and also ourselves in the past, but it is a moot point whether an adequate search for a focus of surface cancer in the excised organ had been made before the cytology result can be justifiably established as being a false positive.

14.3   Screening for cancer of the stomach

This is well established in Japan with its high incidence of disease (Shida, 1971; Takahashi, 1971; Aikawa, 1975) though the logic and approach do seem to emphasize the use of double contrast X-ray more than cytology as an initial technique (Husain, 1976). The opportunity of achieving a higher proportion of early surface cancers does relate to an increased search of symptomatic patients by improved diagnostic methods (Miller and Kaufmann, 1975; Elster *et al.*, 1975; Fevre *et al.*, 1976; Machado *et al.*, 1976; Evans *et al.*, 1978). For example, in the latter series following the introduction of endoscopy the rate of diagnosis of surface cancers went up from 0.5 to 10.0%. Again, in a series from the Massachusetts General Hospital the application of routine gastric cytology on patients attending the gastrointestinal unit resulted in a detection of 8 per 1000 cases of early subclinical cancers of the stomach over and above those diagnosed clinically by other techniques (Husain, 1976).

The most glaring contrast is seen between the Japanese statistics and the four-year survival rate of only 9% in a series from seven countries in Europe (Lundh *et al.*, 1974) where all patients presented with clinical symptoms, the predominant ones being weight loss, pain, vomiting, anorexia and weakness, and with the diagnosis confirmed by barium meal in 96%, gastroscopy in 28% and cytology in less than 6%. This contrasts with Shida's (1971) figures where the mean five-year survival rate was 90% when the tumour was restricted to the mucosa and submucosa, 77% when muscle was invaded and 27% where tumours had reached the serosa. This success is claimed to be due largely to early detection by screening.

The question of whether some form of screening could be afforded in the so-called low incidence countries such as the United States of America or the United Kingdom has been considered in relation to costs (Husain, 1976) and discussed in a *Lancet* leader (1978). The latter noted that even with screening it was found that a mean time of seven months existed between first symptoms and operation (Lundh *et al.*, 1974; Cohn, 1978).

It is obvious that though cytology is beginning to improve in European centres, the pursuit of double contrast X-rays, so vital to initial scanning, has not substantially developed in the United Kingdom as an application in this field.

In Takahashi's (1971) screening programme which reflects the logistics of the Japanese experience, for every 1000 persons seen in the travelling caravan who are initially screened by a personal interview and double contrast fluoroscopy, around 200 to 300 demonstrate sufficient abnormality to pass to the next stage clinic where endoscopy, biopsy and cytology narrow the problem cases down to 50 to 100 persons, consisting of cancers, ulcers, polyps and other pathology.

With the current cost of gastroscopy between £30 to £50, and laboratory examination £15 to £20, and even a gastric wash cytology not less than £20, the application of widespread population screening is not possible. If, however, a greater degree of gastroscopy and double contrast X-ray were to be undertaken on those with symptoms relating to dyspepsia (which would include those suffering from chronic atrophic gastritis, in which more than 75% of cancer develops) then some inroad could be made. However, it is estimated by Barnes *et al.* (1974) that there are about 4500 dyspeptics in every 300 000 population, that is, those served by a District General Hospital. Many are probably over 45 years of age and a method of pre-selection may well have to be more searching and simple to be economic.

It is more than likely that primary screening by cytology or even double contrast X-ray is not going to be cost-effective, especially in low-risk countries, and that some other technique, both simple and economic, may need to be devised as a pre-screening test to provide a group for the more specific radiological and gastroscopic investigations (Husain *et al.*, 1980).

References

Aikawa, K. (1975), Gastric cancer screening in Osaka. *Prev. Med.*, **4**, 154–162.
Barnes, R. J., Gear, M. W. L., Nicol, A. and Dew, A. B. (1974), Study of dyspepsia

in general practice as assessed by endoscopy and radiology. *Br. Med. J.*, **4**, 214–216.

Bemvenuti, G. A., Hattori, K., Levin, B. *et al.* (1975), Endoscopic sampling for tissue diagnosis in gastrointestinal malignancy. *Gastrointest. Endosc.*, **21**, 159–161.

Berg, J. W. (1955), Oesophageal herpes: a complication of cancer therapy. *Cancer*, **8**, 731–740.

Blendis, L. M., Beilby, J. O. W., Wilson, J. P. *et al.* (1967), Carcinoma of the stomach: evaluation of individual and combined diagnostic accuracy of radiology, cytology and gastro-photography. *Br. Med. J.*, **1**, 656–659.

Boddington, M. M. (1978), Cytological aspects. In *Topics in Gastroenterology*, vol. 6, (eds S. C. Truelove and M. R. Heyworth), Blackwell, Oxford, pp. 165–178.

Cabre-Fiol, V., Olo-Garcia, R. and Vilardell, F. (1959), Five years of cytological diagnosis of gastric cancer by 'exfoliative biopsy'. *Proceedings of World Congress of Gastroenterology*, Washington, Williams and Wilkins, Baltimore, p. 1006.

Cabre-Fiol, V., Vilardell, F., Sala-Cladera, E. and Perez Mota, A. (1975), Preoperative cytological diagnosis of gastric leiomyosarcoma. *Gastroenterology*, **68**, 563–566.

Cohn, I. (1978), Gastrointestinal cancer. Surgical survey of abdominal tragedy. *Am. J. Surg.*, **135**, 3–11.

Crozier, R. E., Middleton, M. and Ross, J. R. (1956), Clinical application of gastric cytology. *N. Engl. J. Med.*, **255**, 1128–1131.

Danno, M. (1976), Statistical criteria for the cytology of gastric cancer. A proposal of distance index. *Acta Cytol.*, **20**, 466–468.

Elster, K., Kolazek, F., Shimamoto, K. and Freitag, H. (1975), Early gastric cancer. Experience in Germany. *Endoscopy*, **7**, 5–10.

Evans, D. M. D., Craven, J. L., Murphy, F. and Cleary, B. K. (1978), Comparison of 'early gastric cancer' in Britain and Japan. *Gut*, **19**, 1–9.

Fevre, D. I., Green, P. H. R., Barratt, P. J. and Nagy, G. S. (1976), Review of five cases of early gastric cancer. *Gut*, **17**, 41–47.

Gephart, T. and Graham, R. M. (1959), The cellular detection of carcinoma of the esophagus. *Surg. Gynecol. Obstet.*, **108**, 75–82.

Graham, R. M., Ulfelder, H. and Green, T. H. (1948), The cytologic method as an aid in the diagnosis of gastric carcinoma. *Surg. Gynecol. Obstet.*, **86**, 257–259.

Halter, F., Witzel, L., Gretillat, P. A. *et al.* (1977), Diagnostic value of biopsy, guided lavage and brush cytology in oesophagogastroscopy. *Am. J. Dig. Dis.*, **22**, 129–131.

Hatfield, A. R. W., Whittaker, R. and Gibbs, D. D. (1974), The collection of pancreatic fluid for cytodiagnosis using a duodenoscope. *Gut*, **15**, 305–307.

Hatfield, A. R. W., Smithies, A., Wilkins, R. and Levi, A. J. (1975), Endoscopic retrograde cholangiopancreatography (ERCP) and pure pancreatic juice cytology. A combined diagnostic approach in pancreatic disease. *Gut*, **16**, 405 (abstract).

Henning, N. and Witte, S. (1970), *Atlas of Gastrointestinal Cytodiagnosis*. Thieme, Stuttgart.

Hughes, H. E., Lee, F. D. and MacKenzie, J. F. (1978), Endoscopic cytology and biopsy in the upper gastrointestinal tract. *Clin. Gastroenterol.*, **7**, 375–396.

Husain, O. A. N. (1976), Cytological screening for cancer of the stomach. *Proc. R. Soc. Med.*, **69**, 489–494.

Husain, O. A. N., Zeegan, R., Parkins, R. A. *et al.* (1980), Cytodiagnosis of gastric cancer. In *Recent Advances in Gastrointestinal Pathology* (ed. R. Wright), W. B. Saunders, London, pp. 241–254.

Kameya, S., Nakamura, S., Mizutani, K. *et al.* (1964), Gastrofibrescope for biopsy. *Gastroenterol. Endosc. (Japanese)*, **6**, 36–40.

Kasugai, T. (1964), Gastric biopsy and cytology by the fibregastroscope. *Gastroenterol. Endosc. (Japanese)*, **6**, 187–190.

Kasugai, T. (1968), Evaluation of gastric lavage cytology under direct vision by the fibergastroscope employing Hanks' solution as a washing solution. *Acta Cytol.*, **12**, 345–351.

Kasugai, T. (1976), Gastrofibrescopic techniques for all collections. In *Compendium on Diagnostic Cytology: Tutorials in Cytology*, vol. IV, No. 1 (eds G. L. Wied, L. G. Koss and J. W. Reagan), Chicago University Press, Illinois, pp. 492–496.

Kasugai, T. and Kobayashi, S. (1974), Evaluation of biopsy and cytology in the diagnosis of gastric cancer. *Am. J. Gastroenterol.*, **62**, 199–203.

Kidokoro, T., Soma, S., Seta, R. *et al.* (1966), Gastric cytology under direct vision with special reference to the suction method. *Jpn. Soc. Clin. Cytol.* **5**, 31.

Kline, T. S. and Goldstein, F. (1974), The role of cytology in the diagnosis of gastric lymphoma. *Am. J. Gastroenterol.*, **62**, 193–198.

Kobayashi, S., Prolla, J. C. and Kirsner, J. B. (1970), Brushing cytology of the esophagus and stomach under direct vision by fiberscopes. *Acta Cytol.*, **14**, 219–223.

Lancet leading article (1978), Screening for gastric cancer in the West. *Lancet*, **i**, 1023–1024.

Lasser, A. (1977), Herpes simplex virus oesophagitis. *Acta Cytol.*, **21**, 301–302.

Liavag, I., Marcussen, J. and Serck-Hanssen, A. (1971), Direct vision brush cytology in the diagnosis of gastric disease. *Acta Chir. Scand.*, **137**, 682–688.

Lundh, G., Burn, J. I., Kolig, G. *et al.* (1974), A co-operative international study of gastric cancer. *Ann. R. Coll. Surg. Engl.*, **54**, 3–12.

MacDonald, W. C., Brandenborg, L. L., Taniguchi, I. *et al.* (1963), Exfoliated cytological screening for gastric cancer. *Cancer*, **27**, 163–169.

MacKenzie, J. F., Rogers, I. M., Moule, B. *et al.* (1977), Comparison of double-contrast radiology, standard radiology, endoscopy, also of histology and cytology in the diagnosis of gastric cancer. *Gut*, **18**, 416 (abstract).

Machado, G., Davies, J. D., Tudway, A. J. C. *et al.* (1976), Superficial cancer of the stomach. *Br. Med. J.*, **2**, 77–79.

Mason, M. K. (1965), Surface carcinoma of the stomach. *Gut*, **6**, 185–193.

Miller, G. and Kaufmann, M. (1975), Das magenfrühkarzinom in Europa. *Dtsch. Med. Wochenschr.*, **100**, 1946–1949.

Nelson, R. S. and Lanza, E. L. (1974), The endoscopic diagnosis of gastric lymphoma. *Gastrointest. Endosc.*, **21**, 66–68.

Papanicolaou, G. N. and Cooper, W. A. (1947), The cytology of the gastric fluid in the diagnosis of carcinoma of the stomach. *J. Natl. Cancer Inst.*, **7**, 357–360.

Posner, G., Lightdale, C. J., Cooper, M. *et al.* (1975), Reappraisal of endoscopic tissue diagnosis in secondary gastric lymphoma. *Gastrointest. Endosc.*, **21**, 123–125.

Prolla, J. C., Kobayashi, S. and Kirsner, J. B. (1969), Gastric cancer: some recent improvements in diagnosis based upon the Japanese experience. *Arch. Int. Med.*, **124**, 238–246.

Prolla, J. C., Reilly, R. W., Kirsner, J. B. and Cockerham, L. (1977), Direct vision endoscopic cytology and biopsy in the diagnosis of oesophageal and gastric tumours. Current experience. *Acta Cytol.*, **21**, 399–402.

Raskin, H. F., Kirsner, J. B. and Palmer, W. L. (1959), Role of exfoliative cytology in the diagnosis of cancer of the digestive tract. *J. Am. Med. Assoc.*, **169**, 789–791.

Richards, W. C. D. and Spriggs, A. I. (1961), Cytology of gastric mucosa. *J. Clin. Pathol.*, **14**, 132–139.

Schade, R. O. K. (1960), *Gastric Cytology*, Edward Arnold, London.

Serck-Hanssen, A., Marcussen, J. and Liavag, I. (1973), *Cancer Detection and Prevention*, (ed. C. Maltoni), proceedings of the Second International Symposium on Cancer Detection and Prevention, Bologna, Excerpta Medica, Amsterdam.

Seybolt, J. F. and Papanicolaou, G. N. (1957), The value of cytology in the diagnosis of gastric cancer. *Gastroenterology*, **33**, 369–377.

Shida, S. (1971), Biopsy smear cytology with the fibregastroscope for direct observation. In *Early Gastric Cancer*, Gann Monograph on Cancer Research, 11 (ed. T. Murakami), University of Tokyo Press, Tokyo, pp. 223–232.

Shida, S. (1976), Gastric cytology. Its evaluation for the diagnosis of early gastric cancer. In *Compendium on Diagnostic Cytology, Tutorial in Cytology* (eds G. L. Wied, L. G. Koss and J. W. Reagan), Chicago University Press, Illinois, pp. 457–467.

Smithies, A., Lovell, D., Hishon, S. *et al.* (1975), Value of brush cytology in diagnosis of gastric cancer. *Br. Med. J.*, **4**, 326.

Taebel, D. W., Prolla, J. C. and Kirsner, J. B. (1965), Exfoliative cytology in the diagnosis of stomach cancer. *Ann. Intern. Med.*, **63**, 1018–1026.

Takahashi, K. (1971), Outline of gastric mass survey by X-ray. In *Early Gastric Cancer*, Gann Monograph on Cancer Research, 11 (ed. T. Murakami), University of Tokyo Press, Tokyo, pp. 21–26.

Tamura, K., Masuzawa, M., Akiyama, T. and Rukui, O. (1977), Touch smear cytology for endoscopic diagnosis of gastric carcinoma. *Am. J. Gastroenterol.*, **67**, 463–467.

Tazaki, Y. (1959), Clinical aspects of gastric carcinoma in Japan. *Proceedings of World Congress of Gastroenterology*, Washington, Williams and Wilkins, Baltimore, p. 1148.

Thompson, H., Hoare, A. M., Dykes, P. W. *et al.* (1977), A prospective randomised trial to compare brush cytology before and after punch biopsy for endoscopic diagnosis of gastric cancer. *Gut*, **18**, 398 (abstract).

Traut, H. F., Rosenthal, M., Harrison, J. T. *et al.* (1952), Evaluation of cytologic diagnosis of gastric cancer. *Surg. Gynecol. Obstet.*, **95**, 709–716.

Winawer, S. J., Posner, G., Lightdale, C. J. *et al.* (1976), Endoscopic diagnosis of advanced gastric cancer. Factors influencing yield. *Gastroenterology*, **69**, 1183–1187.

Witte, S. (1959), Die zytodiagnostik des magen karzinomas. *Krebsarzt*, **14**, 408–411.

Witzel, L., Halter, F., Gretillat, P. A. *et al.* (1976), Evaluation of specific value of endoscopic biopsies and brush cytology for malignancies of the oesophagus and stomach. *Gut*, **17**, 375–377.

Wright, S. G., Tomkins, A. M. and Ridley, D. S. (1977), Giardiasis: clinical and therapeutic aspects. *Gut*, **18**, 343–350.

Yoshii, Y., Takanashi, J., Yamaoka, Y. and Kasugai, T. (1970), Significance of imprint smears in cytologic diagnosis of malignant tumours of stomach. *Acta Cytol.*, **14**, 249–253.

Young, J. A. and Hughes, H. E. (1977), Report on a three-year trial of endoscopic cytology of stomach and duodenum. Seventh European Congress of Cytology, Liege.

Index